T0322745

UPCYCLED
BEAUTY

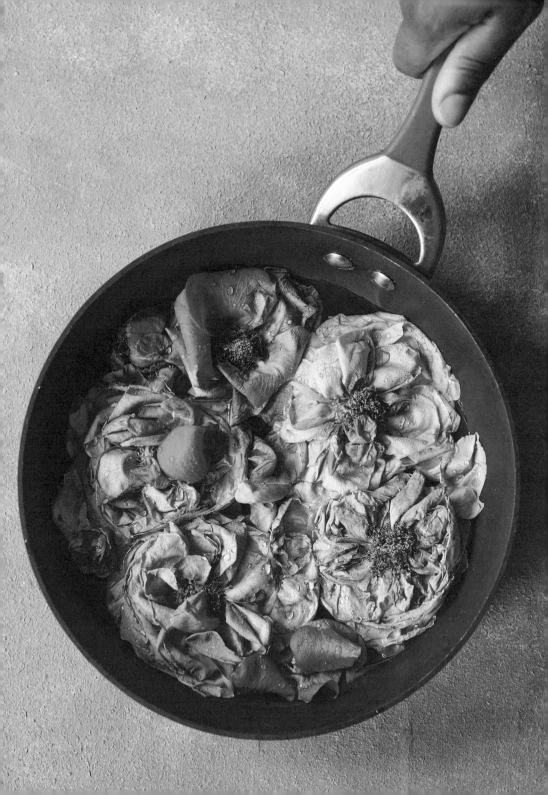

UPCYCLED BEAUTY

Transform everyday
ingredients into no-waste
beauty products

ANNA BRIGHTMAN

PHOTOGRAPHY BY LIZZIE MAYSON

Hardie Grant

BOOKS

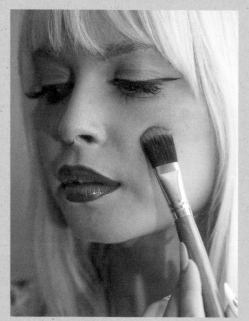
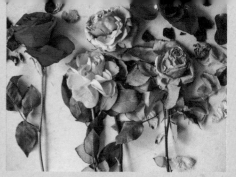
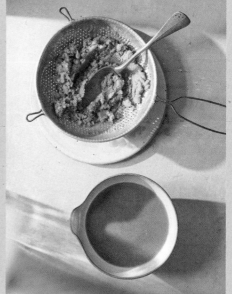
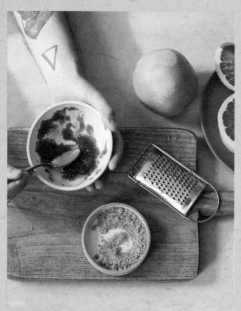
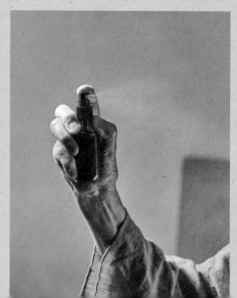

CONTENTS

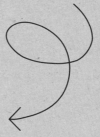

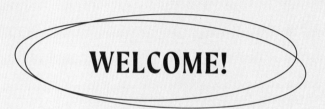

WELCOME!

Hi, and welcome to this book of skincare, beauty and home projects made from upcycled ingredients! I'm Anna - co-founder of UpCircle, a beauty brand my brother William and I started in 2016.

Stuck in jobs we weren't feeling fulfilled in, we wanted to create our own business that would do genuine good for people and planet – something different, something uplifting and something that could represent the future of its industry. So we began looking for our 'penny drop' moment that would play to our different strengths – my experience in fashion PR, supermarket management and my long-term passion for make-up, and William's knowledge in finance.

FINDING THE PROBLEM

On his way to work, William would always stop at a café to pick up a coffee. Out of curiosity, and in the spirit of looking for inspiration wherever it may come, he asked the barista what happened to the used coffee grounds after every single cup of coffee that's made. The answer shocked him. This small independent café produced so many coffee grounds per day that they had to pay the local council to collect and dispose of them. And where did they go? You guessed it, landfill.

FINDING THE SOLUTION

All of a sudden, we had the problem we wanted to tackle: the issue of industry-disposed coffee waste. But what would be our solution? We did as much research on coffee as we possibly could and then began reaching out to coffee shops to see if they'd be willing to let us collect their coffee – a mutually beneficial arrangement: they'd save on disposal costs; we'd get our core ingredient.

As a teenager, my dream job was to be a make-up artist – I'd spend hours watching YouTube tutorials. One of the first lessons you learn is that what comes before great make-up is great skincare. Was it too ambitious to think that we could create a beauty brand on the foundation of circular economy principles and reimagining our perception of waste?

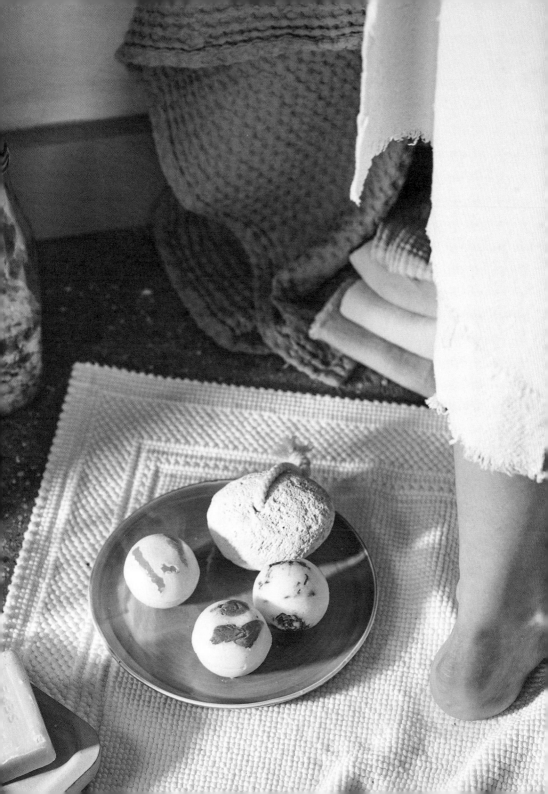

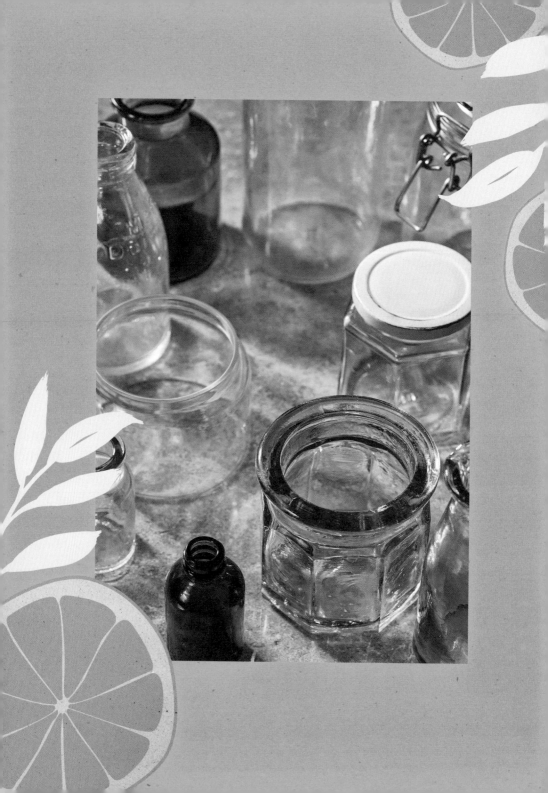

STARTING OUT

Before we knew it, we had a roster of around 100 restaurants, cafés and bars, all within a one-mile radius, from whom we would collect used coffee grounds each day. So we started our upcycled skincare business by making coffee scrubs! We focused on coffee for the first year or so, making a fantastic signature range, but it wasn't long before people caught wind of what we were up to and began approaching us, 'Hey, I own a brand that makes X, but it leaves behind Y. I have no use for Y in what I create, but it's such a shame to throw it away when it still has so much to offer. Do you think you could make use of it at UpCircle?'

When this happens, the first thing we do is establish that the by-product in question has proven skin or hair benefits and would be safe for use in a skin, beauty or haircare product. Next, we must ensure that we would be able to guarantee a reliable supply of this ingredient. Lastly, we need to be able to track it right back to the start of its first life to make sure it's been produced ethically and responsibly from day one. Once this is confirmed, we have samples sent, and the product-development process begins! In this book, I have shared several of the origin stories of ingredients we work with.

CIRCULAR THROUGH AND THROUGH

We rescue countless ingredients to make the UpCircle range. There are those that give a physical texture, like chai spices, coffee grounds and rose petals; there are powders created from olive stones, oat husks, argan shells and apricot kernels; there are residual fruit waters that are evaporated off in the process of making juice concentrates; there are extracted oils, like raspberry, blueberry and date seed extract that are left over from the production of pulps and spreads in the food industry; there are waxes made from fruit peels; there are even upcycled wood extracts like maple bark and cedarwood, which are by-products of the furniture industry.

In this book, we're sharing some of the exact recipes we use, alongside a handful of new ideas and products that just don't have the shelf-life we'd need to make them on a large-scale. I hope this enables you to share in the joy and creativity of the rescue and reuse process. Within these pages, you'll discover the basics of creating skincare from beautiful, skin-loving by-product ingredients, which I hope you'll build on to create your very own skincare favourites. We'd love to see your creations, so please do tag us on social media or email us some photos!

Experiment, get messy and enjoy finding beauty in everything.

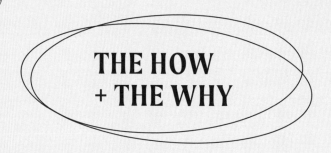

THE HOW
+ THE WHY

Our kitchens are full of ingredients with untapped potential:

An overripe banana can become a breakout-busting face mask (see page 22), and its peel can become a foot mask (see page 26). Wilting herbs can become a lip balm (see page 30) or body butter bars (see page 36) or hair oil (see page 62); and the rinds of your watermelon can transform into a soothing aftersun (see page 38). Of course we have included our signature coffee scrubs – one for body (see page 44) and one for face (see page 46) – but also oat scrubs (see pages 49 and 50). There are many uses for citrus peels – body oil (see page 66), lip scrub (see page 51), bath bombs (see page 98) or surface-cleaning spray (see page 108); and sad-looking flowers can become bath salts (see page 96). The opportunities are endless, but we've consolidated our favourite 50+ projects for you to try.

We'll be making some infused oils – don't worry, it's easier than it sounds – out of would-be-wasted ingredients, to give them a new lease of life. You'll find most of these on pages 132–137.

You'll just need the utensils you have for cooking at home, and most of the ingredients you'll use to make your products will be in your cupboard or fridge already, apart from a few of the more beauty-focused ingredients, but you can find these easily online.

If you're passionate about feeding your skin nourishing products, and about doing a bit more to reduce food waste, I hope this book will become your go-to guide to making products for yourself and your lucky loved-ones!

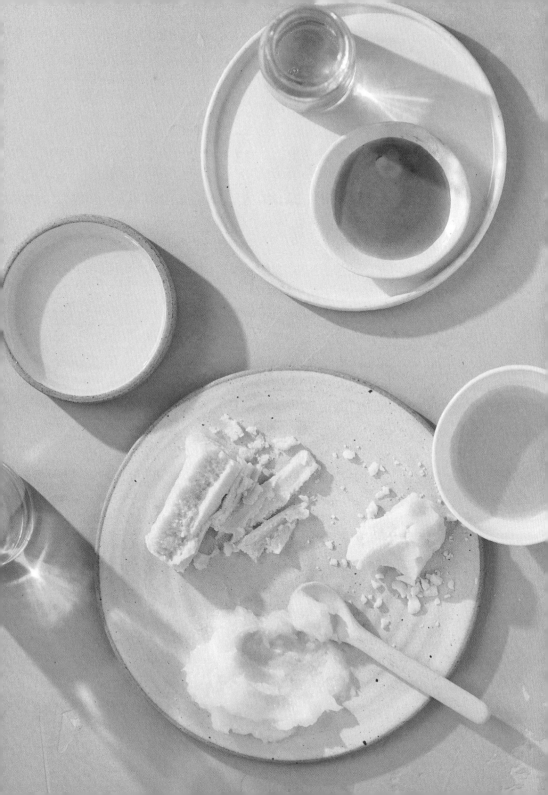

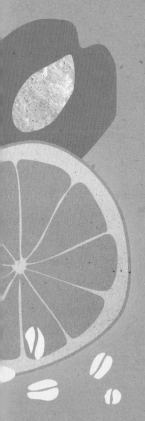

SKIN-LOVING
UPCYCLED INGREDIENTS

**THESE ARE THE INGREDIENTS WE'LL BE TRANSFORMING –
WE WANT YOU TO KNOW WHY THEY'RE SO GREAT!**

- **Apple** – Increases the rate of cellular turnover, helping to keep skin looking and feeling fresh and healthy. High in vitamins A, B and C.

- **Apricot** – Great for firming and strengthening the skin. It contains natural linoleic acid (omega 6), which strengthens the skin's barrier function, as well as oleic acid (omega 9), which softens skin.

- **Avocado** – Great for overall skin health. It's good for hydrating the skin and improving skin elasticity. This is because it helps skin to retain moisture, leaving it feeling nourished and supple.

- **Banana** – Rich in zinc, which can help speed up the healing process and reduce inflammation. Bananas are also chock-full of vitamins and minerals that nourish and revitalise dry, lacklustre skin.

- **Beetroot** – Most useful as a natural pigment. Beetroot can be dried and powdered for use in powdered cosmetics like blusher or eye shadow (see page 87), or added to water to make fabric dye (see page 122).

- **Berries** – Antioxidant-rich! Antioxidants help fight free radicals, which cause early signs of ageing like fine lines. Berries are also packed with vitamins.

- **Citrus fruit** – High in vitamin C, and can help protect the skin from the dulling effects of pollution. They're also antibacterial, which can help to prevent breakouts and hyperpigmentation.

- **Coconut milk** – A nourishing ingredient that works wonders for dry skin conditions such as eczema, dermatitis and psoriasis. The fact that it's a natural fatty acid makes it equally beneficial for your hair and scalp.

- **Coffee** – A gentle natural exfoliator that can be used to buff away dead and dry skin cells. The level of antioxidants has also been proven to increase through the brewing process! Caffeine stimulates blood flow, which is why coffee also has a brightening effect on dull skin.

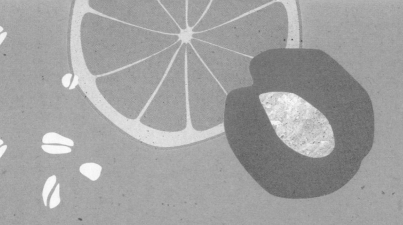

- **Cucumber** – Filled with many essential nutrients, minerals and antioxidants, which is why it helps with clogged and visibly enlarged pores. Cucumber can also help to combat both excessive oiliness and dryness.

- **Flowers** – Soothing and gentle, flowers work wonders on sensitive skin. They smell great and have an uplifting effect on both skin and mood!

- **Ginger** – Great for reducing redness and puffiness. It contains compounds that can stimulate collagen production and thus help to keep the skin looking healthy and glowing.

- **Herbs** – Fantastic for regulating sebum production, which helps control oily skin. This is why herbs are often top ingredients in spot and acne treatments.

- **Oats** – Contain polysaccharides, which have a hydrating effect and support skin-barrier function. They also work well as a gently cleansing natural exfoliator.

- **Potato** – Contains antioxidants and glow-inducing vitamins A, B and C. Potatoes also contain an enzyme called catecholase, which is helpful in reducing dark spots and evening out skin tone.

- **Pumpkin** – High in vitamin A and salicylic acid, which is great for blemish-prone skin, as well as beta-carotene, which helps reduce the appearance of dark spots.

- **Chai spices** – As well as smelling incredible, spices are also good for boosting circulation, helping skin to appear bright and well rested.

- **Watermelon** – Helps skin to appear more radiant. Watermelon contains vitamins such as A, B and C, which work together to nourish, soothe and protect your skin.

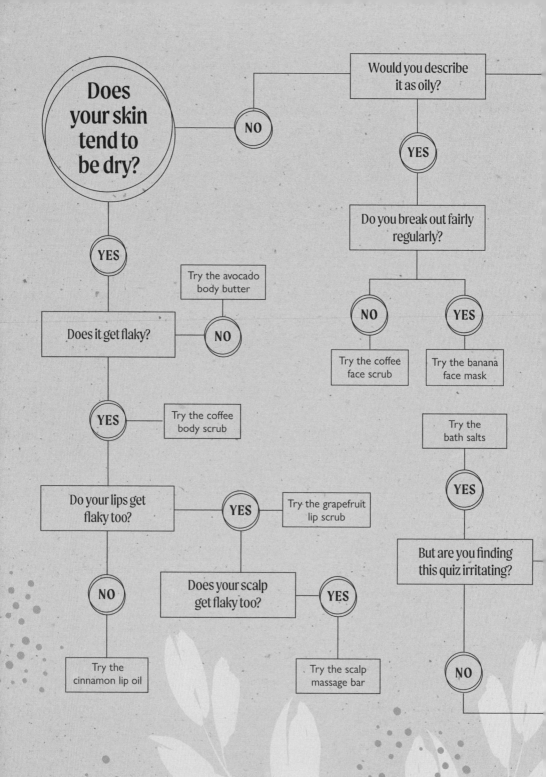

Does your skin tend to be dry?

NO → Would you describe it as oily?

YES → Do you break out fairly regularly?

NO → Try the coffee face scrub

YES → Try the banana face mask

YES →

Does it get flaky?

NO → Try the avocado body butter

YES → Try the coffee body scrub

Do your lips get flaky too?

YES → Try the grapefruit lip scrub

NO → Try the cinnamon lip oil

Does your scalp get flaky too?

YES → Try the scalp massage bar

Try the bath salts

YES →

But are you finding this quiz irritating?

NO →

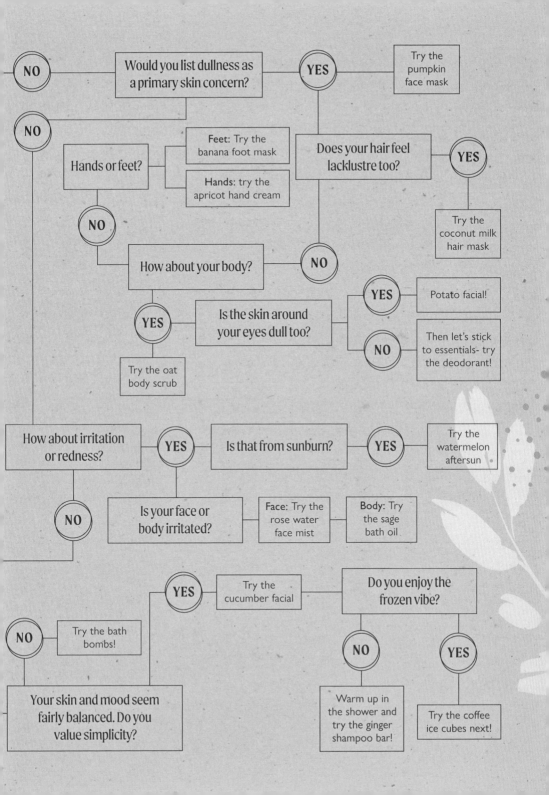

NO — Would you list dullness as a primary skin concern? — **YES** — Try the pumpkin face mask

NO

Hands or feet? — Feet: Try the banana foot mask

Hands: try the apricot hand cream

Does your hair feel lacklustre too? — **YES**

Try the coconut milk hair mask

NO

How about your body? — **NO**

YES — Is the skin around your eyes dull too? — **YES** — Potato facial!

NO — Then let's stick to essentials- try the deodorant!

Try the oat body scrub

How about irritation or redness? — **YES** — Is that from sunburn? — **YES** — Try the watermelon aftersun

NO

Is your face or body irritated? — Face: Try the rose water face mist — Body: Try the sage bath oil

YES — Try the cucumber facial — Do you enjoy the frozen vibe?

NO — Try the bath bombs!

Your skin and mood seem fairly balanced. Do you value simplicity?

NO — Warm up in the shower and try the ginger shampoo bar!

YES — Try the coffee ice cubes next!

MASKS

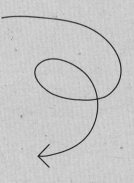

In a fast-paced world where stress and pollution abound, our skin often bears the brunt of our daily challenges. A face mask helps to slow things down, giving our skin – and our minds – a moment to restore and replenish. The canvas is your face, and the palette is an abundant array of simple natural ingredients that cater to your unique skin type and specific concerns, be it soothing sensitivity, combating acne or rejuvenating tired skin.

Before applying any mask, make sure your skin, heels or hair are cleansed first.

If there are any leftovers of any of these masks, you can store them in a reusable container in the fridge for up to 3 days. However, using the mask immediately after preparation is recommended for maximum freshness and effectiveness.

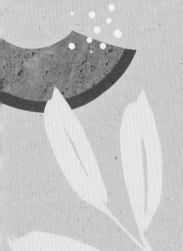

REJUVENATING
AVOCADO FACE MASK

MAKES 2 MASKS

INGREDIENTS:

1 overripe avocado
1 tablespoon oat flour *(you can make your own by blending oats to a fine powder in a blender)*
1 teaspoon almond oil, or any other plant-based oil
1 teaspoon agave syrup *(optional, for extra hydration)*
2–3 drops of lavender essential oil *(optional, for a soothing aroma)*

TIP:

If you're looking for a use for the avocado stone or the skins, try the Avocado Cuticle Oil on page 60.

Getting a perfectly ripe avocado every time is a skill I do not possess. If you ever leave it too long, or realise you've got an avocado browning at the bottom of a fruit bowl that you're not so keen to eat, then use it as a face mask instead. The avocado is a powerhouse of essential nutrients and natural oils that can deeply nourish and revitalise your skin.

01 Scoop out the flesh of your overripe avocado into a mixing bowl. Mash thoroughly with a fork or the back of a spoon until you achieve a smooth, lump-free consistency. Add the oat flour and almond oil, along with the agave syrup and lavender essential oil (if using).

02 Stir all the ingredients together until well combined. The mixture should form a thick, creamy paste that's easy to apply to your face.

03 Before applying the face mask, cleanse your face with a gentle cleanser to remove any make-up, dirt, or impurities.

04 Using clean fingers or a face mask brush, apply an even layer of the mask to your face, avoiding the delicate area around the eyes. Once the face mask is applied, relax and allow the mask to work its magic for about 15–20 minutes to deeply nourish your skin.

05 Gently rinse off the mask with warm water. Pat dry with a soft towel and follow up with a moisturiser.

06 If you haven't used this all up immediately, it can be stored in the fridge in an air-tight container to be used within 3 days.

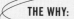

THE WHY:

- Avocado is rich in healthy fats, such as omega-3 fatty acids and oleic acid, which help to moisturise and hydrate the skin, leaving it soft and supple. The almond oil offers added nourishment and moisture.

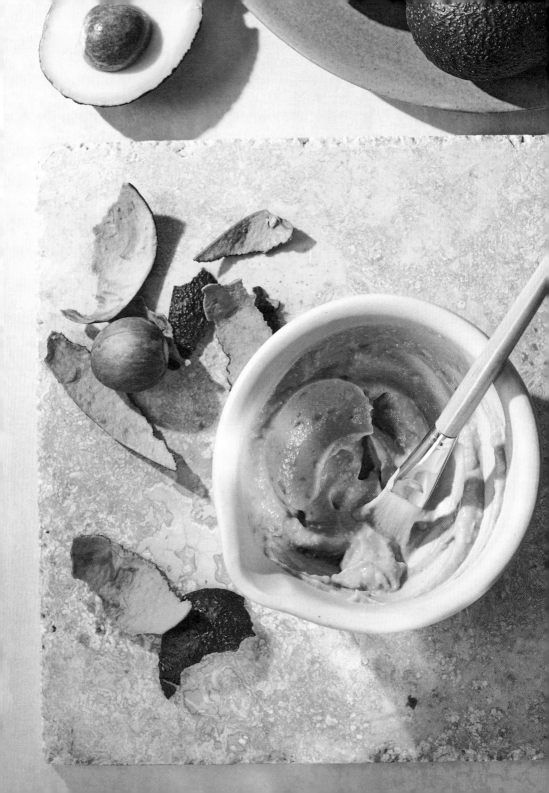

COLLAGEN-BOOSTING PUMPKIN FACE MASK

MAKES 2 MASKS

INGREDIENTS:

approx. 50 g *(2 oz)* leftover
   pumpkin carvings and pulp
1 tablespoon melted coconut oil
pinch of ground cinnamon,
   or a small glug of maple syrup
   (optional)

Halloween is my favourite night of the year. As a teenager, my dream job was to be a make-up artist, and it was this dream that first developed my keen interest in skincare. As they always say, the best make-up starts with great skincare.

All the face paint, sugar-laden goodies and repetitive grimacing at Halloween can easily leave your skin looking a little worse for wear the next day. This mask will bring life back into your zombified flesh!

I'm a big fan of pumpkin carving. What I love a lot less is the wastefulness of chucking away all the pumpkin flesh and the parts I've cut away. Yes, pumpkin soup, pumpkin pie and pumpkin skin crisps are DELICIOUS, but so is a pumpkin face mask! I also tend to find pumpkins sold specifically for carving aren't the most tasty, so this is perfect for the carved-out flesh.

01 Simply whack everything into a blender and blitz to combine. Once smooth, decant into a bowl, then apply to a clean, dry face using clean fingers or a face mask brush, avoiding the delicate area around the eyes.

02 Sit back and relax for 10–15 minutes, then wash off with warm water and a soft cloth before patting your face dry.

03 If you haven't used this all up immediately, it can be stored in the fridge in an air-tight container to be used within 3 days.

THE WHY:

- Pumpkin gets its famous sunset hue from a pigment called beta-carotene (also found in carrots), which is absorbed through the skin and turned into vitamin A by the body. This helps with forming collagen, a major component in healthy skin. Pumpkin is full of antioxidants like vitamin C, which helps to soften and soothe dry skin. If you're anything like me, then your skin will probably appreciate this the day after it's had a night caked in extremely ghoulish make-up and/or glitter!

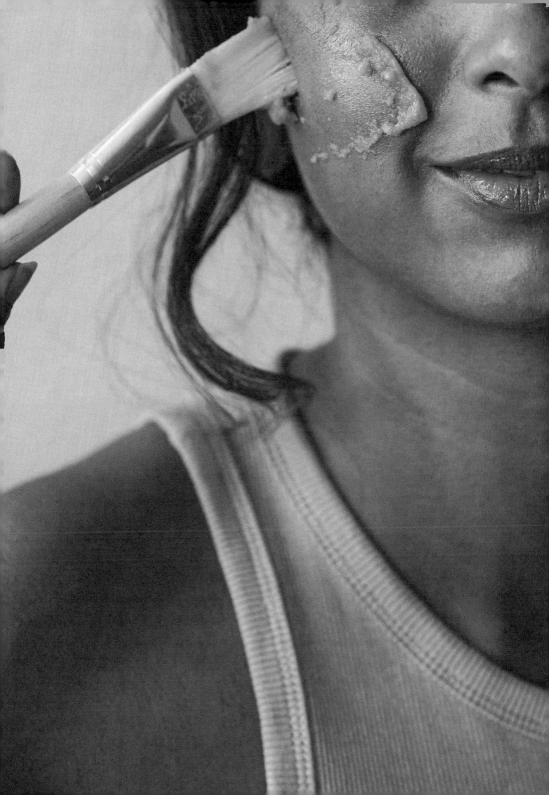

BREAKOUT-BUSTING BANANA FACE MASK

MAKES 2 MASKS

INGREDIENTS:

1 overripe banana
1 tablespoon almond flour, *or oat flour if you need a nut-free option*
1 teaspoon melted coconut oil
1 teaspoon maple syrup
2-3 drops of chamomile essential oil

TIP:
Feet: Try the banana foot mask (see page 26).

The method and application process for this mask are identical to the Rejuvenating Avocado Face Mask on page 18, but this one has its own unique skin benefits. It's a great way to use up a banana that's just too soft and squishy to eat. And if you want to use up the banana peel, too, try the foot mask on page 26.

01 Peel your banana and thoroughly mash the fruit in a mixing bowl until you achieve a smooth, lump-free consistency. Add the almond flour and coconut oil, along with the chamomile essential oil.

02 Stir until well-combined and it's a thick, creamy paste that's easy to apply to your face.

03 Before applying the face mask, cleanse your face to remove any make-up, dirt, or impurities.

04 Using clean fingers or a face mask brush, apply an even layer of the mask to your face, avoiding the delicate area around the eyes. Once applied, relax and allow the mask to work its magic for about 15–20 minutes.

05 Gently rinse off the mask with warm water. Pat dry with a soft towel and follow up with a moisturiser.

06 If you haven't used this all up immediately, store in the fridge in an air-tight container to be used within 3 days.

THE WHY:

• Overripe bananas are rich in natural oils and potassium, providing deep hydration to dry and dull skin, leaving it feeling soft and supple. Bananas also contain vitamins A and C, which are essential for healthy skin: vitamin A can help reduce fine lines, while vitamin C can help brighten and even out your skin tone. In addition, bananas are rich in vitamin B6, which can help regulate the hormones that cause acne and reduce inflammation in the skin.

• As an added bonus, chamomile is a hero oil that helps to soothe and calm irritated skin, reducing the redness and sensitivity that often come with a bout of acne or spots.

POTATO FACIAL

INGREDIENTS:

a piece of raw potato *(that's it!)*

TIP:

I know cucumber slices are what you usually see depicted over people's eyes during a facial, but potato slices work just as well. They're excellent at soothing under-eye puffiness and helping to reduce the appearance of dark circles.

If you've got half a potato left over from cooking, don't throw it away. A potato facial might sound odd, but trust me. The potato acts almost like a facial massage bar or gua sha stone, but has added benefits, like soothing inflamed or sunburned skin. This is a lot like the Cucumber Facial on page 77, which uses a frozen cucumber to similar effect.

01 It's pretty simple, to be honest! After cleansing your skin, rub the cut part of the potato across your skin in circular motions, or follow the sort of facial massage routine you might use with a gua sha stone (give this a quick google if needs be, there are thousands of 'how to' videos online).

02 The edge of the potato that you're rubbing onto your skin should be moist, so if it's dried out, cut off a thin slice before you begin. There shouldn't be any friction between the potato and your skin.

03 Continue for as long as you like and then leave the potato juice to soak in for 10–20 minutes before washing off with warm water. Pat your skin dry with a clean towel.

04 If you haven't used this all up immediately, it can be stored in the fridge in an air-tight container to be used within 3 days.

THE WHY:

Potato is a great moisturising ingredient. It contains hyaluronic acid, which is naturally produced by your own skin. It's packed with vitamins and nutrients that nourish and hydrate the skin, leaving it feeling supple and bouncy. It's also great at preventing acne and helping to soothe acne-inflamed skin, and studies suggest that potatoes are effective at helping to minimise early signs of ageing because they contain antioxidants and glow-inducing vitamins A, B and C, which can help to improve skin elasticity and fullness. The act of massaging the potato into your skin also improves blood flow, making your skin look brighter and more well-rested.

CONDITIONING COCONUT MILK HAIR MASK
for healthy shine

MAKES 2 MASKS
*for mid-long-length hair,
more for short hair*

INGREDIENTS:

about 120 ml *(4 fl oz/½ cup)*
  coconut milk *(or however much
  you have)*
2 tablespoons melted coconut oil
  *(add another 1 tablespoon if your
  hair is very dry)*
5-6 drops of rosemary essential oil
1 tablespoon agave syrup

OPTIONAL EXTRAS:
*(depending on your hair's
specific needs)*

1 tablespoon castor oil
  (for damaged hair)
1 tablespoon argan oil *(for dandruff/
  flaky scalp)*
1 tablespoon olive oil *(for brittle hair
  and split ends)*
1 tablespoon aloe vera gel *(for an
  irritated scalp) –* see page 139
  for how to extract aloe gel
  from a leaf

I use coconut milk in so many things – curries, desserts, smoothies. Tins of coconut milk are a food-cupboard staple for me, but a can is usually more than what I need in recipes, meaning that I often end up with about a third of a can left over. If I'm all smoothied out, then I use that last bit for this instead. The rosemary essential oil is great for hair growth. If you like, you can make your own herbal hair oil instead using the recipe on page 62.

01 In a mixing bowl, combine the coconut milk, melted coconut oil, rosemary oil and agave syrup, along with any extras you are including. Stir the mixture well until all the ingredients are fully incorporated.

02 Comb or brush your hair to remove any tangles and dampen it slightly with water. Divide into sections.

03 Apply the hair mask generously from the roots to the ends, covering all areas. Gently massage the mask into your scalp to promote blood circulation. You may wish to secure your hair with a clip or hair tie, or wrap your hair with a shower cap, a towel or a wax wrap.

04 Leave the mask on for about an hour, allowing it to deeply penetrate and nourish your hair. The longer you leave it on, the more time the coconut milk will have to work its magic.

05 When you're ready, remove the wrapping and rinse off the hair mask with cool or lukewarm water. Follow up with a gentle and eco-friendly shampoo and conditioner to remove any excess oils and to ensure your hair is clean and fresh.

06 If you haven't used this all up immediately, it can be stored in the fridge in an air-tight container to be used within 3 days.

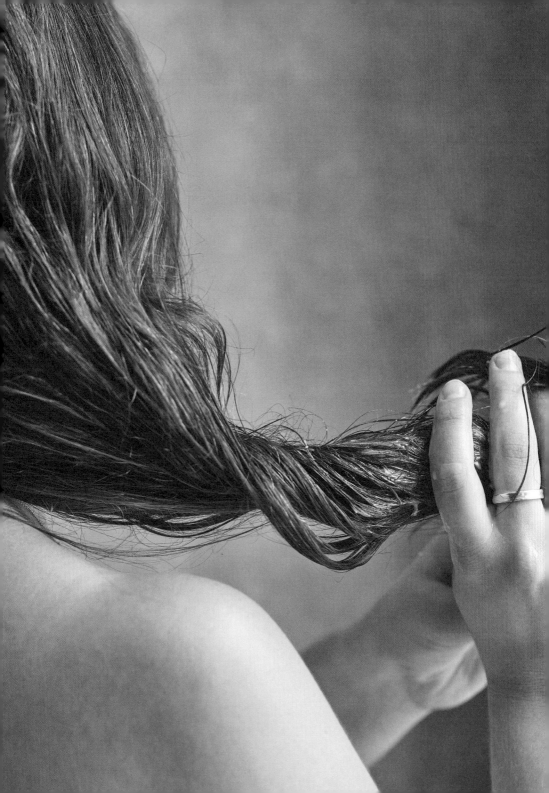

SOFTENING BANANA PEEL FOOT MASK

**MAKES ENOUGH
FOR 3 TREATMENTS**

INGREDIENTS:

2 banana peels – the riper
the bananas, the more
moisturising they'll be!
1 tablespoon coconut oil
1 tablespoon olive oil
1 tablespoon oat flour *(you can
make your own by blending
oats to a fine powder)*
1 teaspoon lemon juice *(optional,
for added exfoliation)*

YOU WILL NEED:

foot file or pumice stone
a pair of thick socks

THE WHY:

• Banana peels are high in vitamins
A, B, C and E, and are amazing
at nourishing dry, sore hands
and cracked heels, promoting
healing and rejuvenation. The
gentle natural enzymes in banana
peels also help to exfoliate dead
skin cells, revealing smoother
and healthier skin underneath.
Better yet, banana peels possess
anti-inflammatory properties
that can aid in reducing the
redness, swelling and discomfort
associated with cracked heels.

Once, while on holiday, I slightly burned the base of my heels on sunbaked tiles. I massaged them with the inside of banana peels before putting on sleep socks. My feet felt so soothed by the morning. If using the peels alone feels a bit tooooo 'zero-waste vibes', have a go at this foot mask recipe. It's not just for burned soles, either – it is a great treatment for dry, cracked heels.

01 Place the banana peels in a blender and blend them until you achieve a smooth, creamy consistency.

02 Transfer the blended banana peels into a mixing bowl and add the coconut oil, olive oil, oat flour and lemon juice (if using). Stir well to form a smooth, thick paste.

03 Next, clean and prep your feet! Wash them thoroughly with warm water and mild soap. Pat dry with a towel and gently remove any dead skin or calluses using a foot file or pumice stone.

04 Take a generous amount of the banana peel foot mask and apply it evenly over your heels and the surrounding areas. Massage the mask into your skin using circular motions to ensure maximum absorption, then put on a pair of thick socks to lock in the moisture and allow the ingredients to work their magic. Leave for at least 30 minutes, or preferably overnight, so the nutrients and moisturising properties can deeply penetrate your skin.

05 When you're ready, remove your socks and wash off the foot mask with warm water. Gently pat your feet dry and apply a natural foot cream or moisturiser.

06 For best results, repeat this foot mask treatment 2–3 times a week until you notice a sustained improvement.

07 If you haven't used this all up immediately, store in the fridge in an air-tight container and use within 3 days.

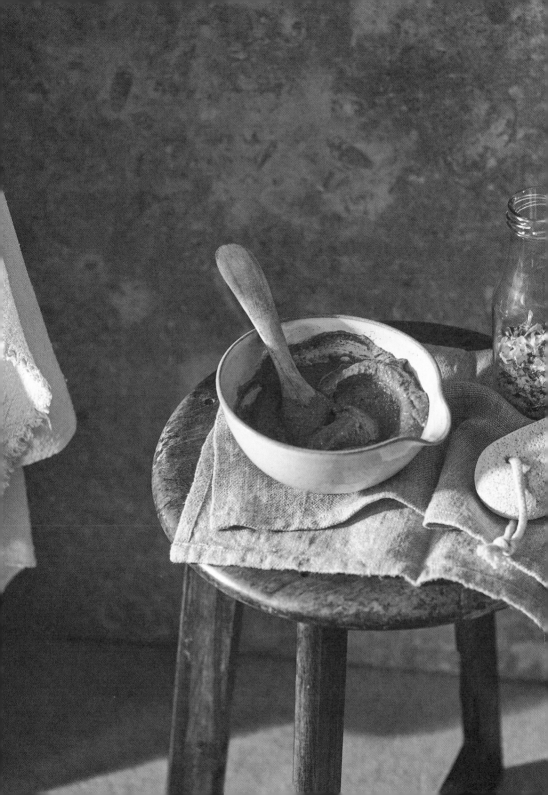

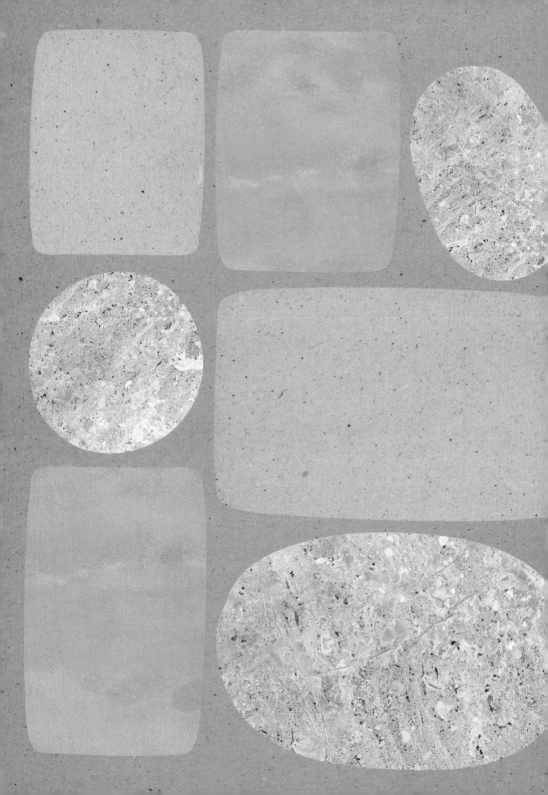

BALMS, BARS + BUTTERS

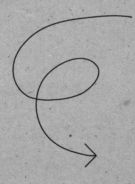

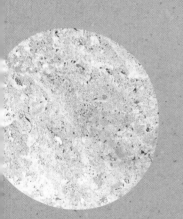

For these recipes you'll be channelling your inner alchemist, crafting nourishing and soothing oil-based skin treats that are a joy both to make and to use. Oil-based skincare lasts significantly longer, so you can enjoy these over months rather than days or weeks. If you're looking for a beautiful gift that the giftee won't need to use in a hurry, then head straight for the 'bars'.

All recipes in this chapter should be stored in a cool, dry place and used within 3 months (unless otherwise specified in the recipe).

WILTED MINT LIP BALM
with homemade mint-infused oil

MAKES 1 POT

INGREDIENTS:

1 tablespoon candelilla wax, or
   another wax of your choice
   (carnauba, candelilla, rice bran,
   berry)
2 tablespoons coconut oil
1 tablespoon shea butter
1 teaspoon almond oil, or other
   carrier oil of your choice (see
   page 102 for suggestions)
4 drops of homemade
   mint-infused oil
   (see page 132)

YOU WILL NEED:

heatproof bowl and saucepan
   to create a bain-marie/
   double-boiler
lip balm containers or small
   reusable tins

TIP:

*If you're not a fan of minty balms
and prefer yours fruitier, you
can use the Orange Peel Oil or
the Lemon Peel Oil on pages
134–135.*

Most of the big brands' lip balms seem to make my lips drier, or I end up feeling like I need to reapply the balm constantly. I'm more into a balm that provides genuine, long-lasting nourishment. Beeswax is an undeniably high-performance base for any balm, but there are several good plant-based alternatives, like carnauba, candelilla, rice bran or berry wax. Any of these can be used to create lip, body or scar-treatment balms. Here, we'll make a mint infusion using up leftover wilted mint leaves, before using it in a delicious and moisturising lip balm.

01 Start by following the instructions on page 132 to make your homemade mint infusion from wilted mint leaves.

02 Fill the saucepan with about 5 cm (2 in) water and bring to a simmer over a medium heat. Place the heatproof bowl on top of the saucepan, ensuring it fits securely without touching the water.

03 Add the candelilla wax, coconut oil, shea butter and almond oil to the heatproof bowl. Stir occasionally until all the ingredients are completely melted and combined. This should take about 5–7 minutes.

04 Finally, add the mint oil and stir.

05 Carefully pour the liquid lip balm into your chosen container and leave to cool and solidify – this usually takes around 1–2 hours. Store in a cool, dry place and use within 3 months.

06 Apply to dry lips as needed!

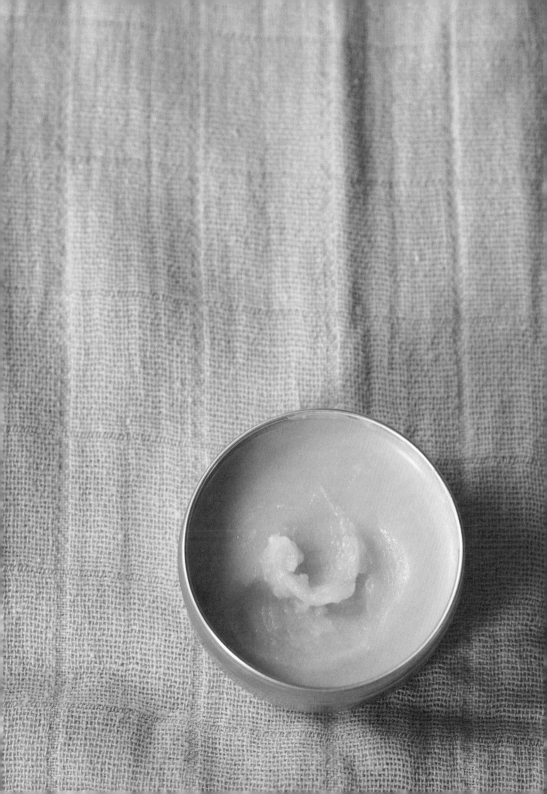

APRICOT HAND CREAM
with homemade apricot kernel oil

MAKES 1 JAR
(approx. 100 ml/3½ fl oz)

INGREDIENTS:

15 drops Apricot Kernel Oil
  (see page 136)
4 tablespoons shea butter
2 tablespoons coconut oil
1 tablespoon candelilla wax, or
  another wax of your choice
  (carnauba, candelilla, rice bran,
  berry)
1 tablespoon vegetable glycerine
5–6 drops of sage oil *(or another
  essential oil of your choice)*

YOU WILL NEED:

heatproof bowl and a saucepan
  to create a bain-marie
  /double-boiler
spatula
small glass jar or tin

The skin on our hands gets a lot of exposure, and in this post-Covid world, it's likely that a lot more serious handwashing is going on. Hands often end up dry, scaly and rough, especially in the colder months. There is an insider secret that you get the best out of a product if you use it regularly and consistently, and this especially holds true for hand creams. For this hand cream, we'll be making an apricot kernel oil first to use in the cream.

01 Start by following the instructions on page 136 to create your homemade apricot kernel oil.

02 Fill a saucepan with about 5 cm (2 in) water and bring to a simmer over a low heat. Place a heatproof bowl on top of the saucepan, ensuring it fits securely without touching the water. Add the shea butter, coconut oil and the wax to the bowl and melt, stirring occasionally, until everything is melted and blended. Remove from the heat and let it cool slightly.

03 Add your homemade apricot kernel oil to the melted mixture, along with the glycerine. Stir well to combine. Add the sage oil and stir once more until the fragrance is evenly distributed throughout the cream.

04 Allow the mixture to cool to room temperature, but don't let it solidify completely. Use a spatula to transfer the semi-solid hand cream into a clean glass jar or tin. Now let the hand cream solidify completely by leaving it undisturbed at room temperature for a few hours or overnight.

05 Your homemade apricot oil hand cream is now ready to use! To do so, apply a small amount to your hands whenever they need an extra dose of nourishment. It will leave your hands feeling soft, smooth and pampered.

06 Store in a cool, dry place and use within 3 months.

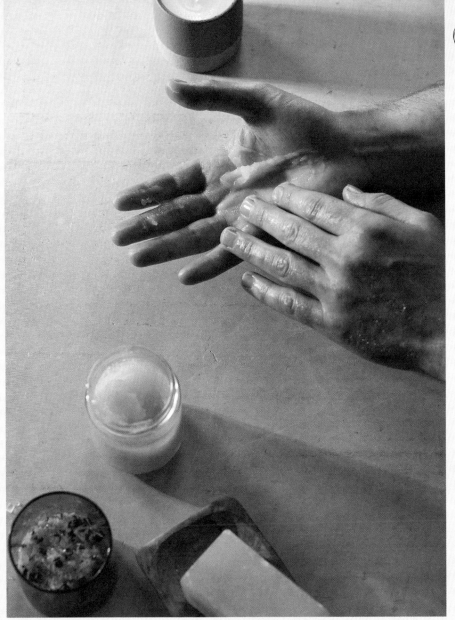

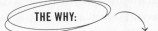
THE WHY:

- The apricot kernel oil contains natural linoleic acid (omega 6), which strengthens the skin's barrier function, and oleic acid (omega 9), which softens skin and gives it a satin-like feel.

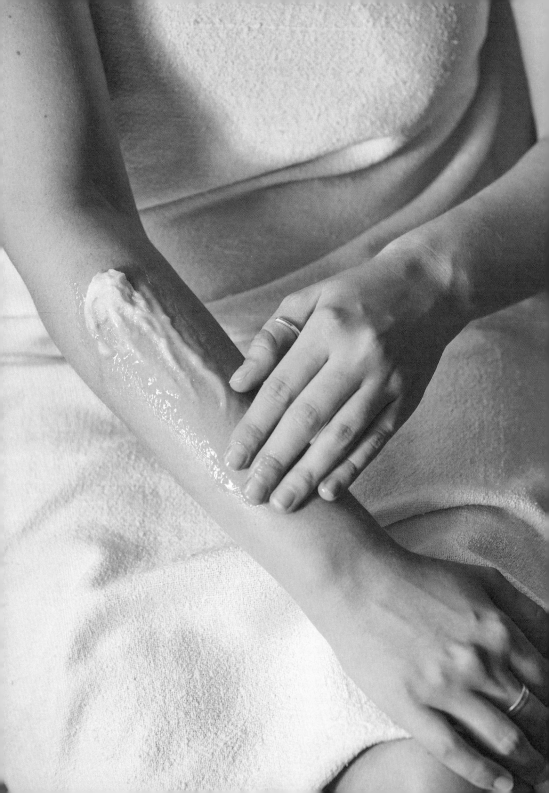

BODY BUTTER
with avocado stone powder

MAKES 1 JAR
(approx. 100 ml/3½ fl oz)

INGREDIENTS:

2–3 avocado stones
2 tablespoons shea butter
1 tablespoon cocoa butter
2 tablespoons almond oil, or any
   other carrier oil of your choice
3 drops of Lemon Peel Oil
   (see page 126)
3 drops of rosemary oil

YOU WILL NEED:

blender and/or pestle and mortar
heatproof bowl and saucepan
   to create a bain-marie
   /double-boiler
glass jar – about the size of a
   small jam jar

The moment of cutting open an avocado is always tense. Will it be underripe, will it be overripe, will the stone be huge, leaving hardly any room for the edible part? It's a gamble! Given that avocado stones will always be a relatively large part of the fruit, you'll be happy to hear that they can be utilised, and they host many skin benefits.

01 Wash and thoroughly dry the avocado stones after eating the fruit. Ideally, leave for 3–4 days to dry out fully.

02 Once dry, crush the stones using a nutcracker or by placing them between two chopping boards and pushing with all your might! Next, pop into a blender and blitz to form a smooth powder. If your blender can't make the powder fine enough, you can transfer to a pestle and mortar at this point and grind by hand. You need 1 tablespoon of this avocado stone powder for the body butter.

03 Fill the saucepan with about 5 cm (2 in) water and bring to a simmer over a medium heat. Place the heatproof bowl on top of the saucepan, ensuring it fits securely without touching the water. Add the shea and cocoa butters and melt, stirring occasionally, until everything is completely melted and blended.

04 Add all three oils and stir, then add your avocado powder and mix thoroughly. Pour the mixture into your container and leave at room temperature until set. Your body butter should keep for about 2 months.

05 To use, apply to clean, dry skin and enjoy the rich nourishment of these skin-loving ingredients!

THE WHY:

• Avocado stones are rich in fatty acids, making them an ideal base for a deeply hydrating skin butter.

BODY BUTTER BARS
with browning or wilted herbs

MAKES 2–3 BARS
*depending on the size
of your mould*

INGREDIENTS:

4 tablespoons cocoa butter
4 tablespoons shea butter
4 tablespoons coconut oil
4 tablespoons sweet almond oil,
    or any other carrier oil of
    your choice (see page 102 for
    suggestions)
1 tablespoon candelilla wax or
    soy wax
10–15 drops of your favourite
    essential oil for fragrance
    *(I like to use a mix of vanilla
    and ylang-ylang here)*
4 tablespoons browning or
    wilted herbs

YOU WILL NEED:

heatproof bowl and saucepan
    to create a bain-marie/
    double-boiler
silicone moulds or an ice cube tray
glass jar or tin

With the simple addition of wax a butter becomes a bar. Deeply hydrating, pleasant to use and travel-friendly, lotion bars are gaining popularity and can be a great plastic-free alternative to bottled lotions and creams.

01 Fill the saucepan with about 5 cm (2 in) water and bring to a simmer over a low heat. Place the heatproof bowl on top of the saucepan, ensuring it fits securely without touching the water. Add the cocoa butter, shea butter and coconut oil to the heatproof bowl. Allow them to melt slowly, stirring occasionally, until completely melted and combined. This usually takes around 5–7 minutes.

02 Remove from the heat and add the almond oil (or your chosen carrier oil) and candelilla or soy wax to the melted mixture. Stir gently until the wax is fully melted and all the ingredients are well combined.

03 At this point, add in your choice of essential oils. Finally, stir in the herbs, mixing well to ensure they are evenly distributed.

04 Carefully pour the liquid body butter mixture into the silicone moulds or ice cube tray. Leave undisturbed at room temperature until the body butter bars have completely cooled and solidified. This process usually takes a few hours, but you can expedite it by placing the moulds in the fridge.

05 Once the body butter bars are fully solid, gently pop them out of the moulds and transfer them to a clean, dry glass jar or tin for storage. Store in a cool, dry place and use within 3 months.

06 To use, simply glide a body butter bar over your skin. The natural heat of your skin will melt a small amount of the butter, leaving your skin feeling moisturised, soft and pampered.

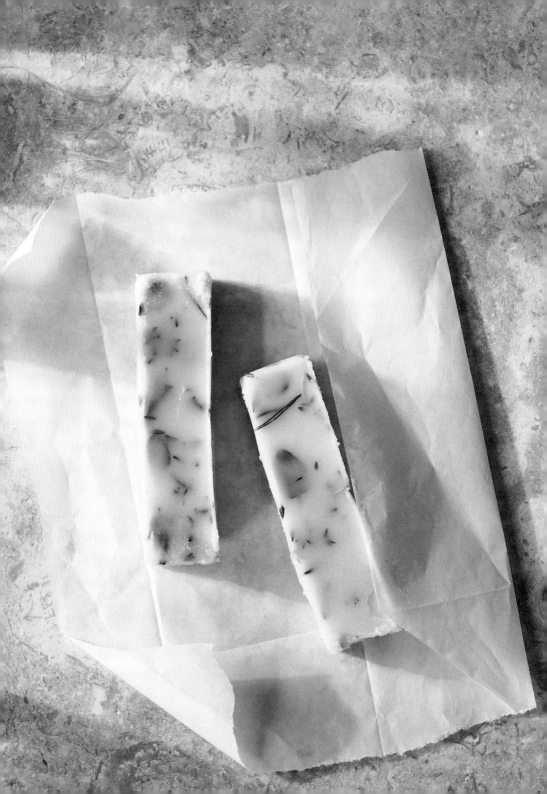

SKIN-SOOTHING AFTERSUN
with watermelon rinds

MAKES 3–4 TREATMENTS
depending on the size of the affected area

INGREDIENTS:

watermelon rinds from a freshly
  cut watermelon, chopped
  into chunks
1 tablespoon aloe vera gel *(see
  page 139 for how to extract aloe
  gel from a leaf)*
1 teaspoon coconut oil
few drops of lavender essential oil

YOU WILL NEED:

blender / food processor
fine-mesh strainer
glass jar or container with a lid
  (like a Kilner jar)

Watermelon is my favourite fruit, no competition. It's hydrating and refreshing to eat, and has the exact same effect when used on the skin. The rinds of watermelon, much like other fruit peels and pith, are packed with vitamins and antioxidants, and have anti-inflammatory properties that can help calm and nourish sun-exposed skin. We've also added some aloe vera gel for its cooling and soothing properties, and some coconut oil for extra moisture. Now, the best course of action is to protect your skin adequately from the sun in the first place and avoid getting burned at all costs. This is just in case you've had a bit of a 'mare...

01 Place the watermelon rind chunks in a blender or food processor and blend until completely puréed. The mixture should have a smooth, gel-like consistency.

02 Using a fine-mesh strainer, strain the watermelon rind purée into a clean bowl. Press down on the purée with a spoon to extract as much liquid as possible.

03 Add the aloe vera gel and coconut oil and stir well to ensure everything is thoroughly combined. Add the lavender essential oil and mix again.

04 Transfer the mixture into a clean glass jar or container with a secure lid. This will keep in the refrigerator for up to 5 days.

05 To use, apply gently and liberally to the affected areas of your skin. Allow the gel to absorb and soothe your skin naturally.

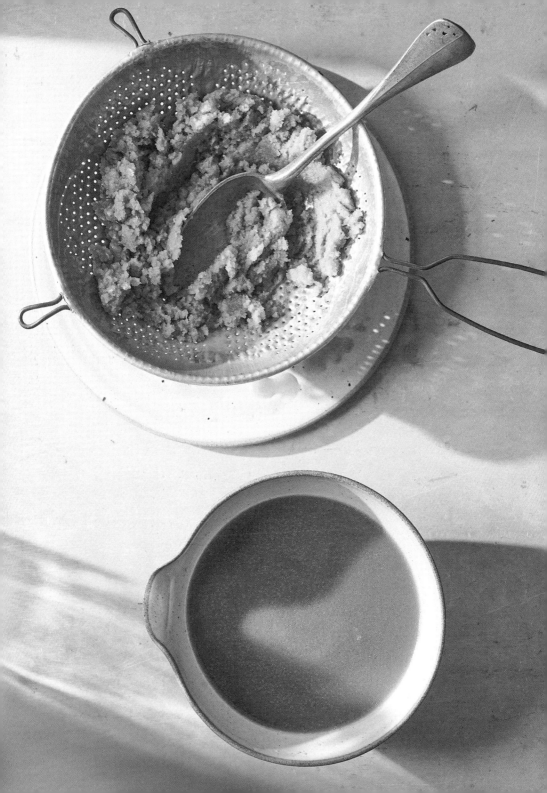

GINGER SHAMPOO BAR

MAKES 2–3 BARS
depending on the size of your mould

INGREDIENTS:

2 tablespoons carnuba wax
10 drops of argan oil
10 drops of Ginger Oil
 (see page 133)
3 tablespoons liquid Castile soap
1 tablespoon apple cider vinegar

YOU WILL NEED:

heatproof bowl and saucepan
 to create a bain-marie/
 double-boiler
soap or shampoo bar mould

TIP:

Make sure your bar is able to drain and dry between uses, if you do you'll get a lot more uses from it.

The average time it takes us to develop a product is about a year, but it took us four to design a shampoo formula we were completely happy with. The manufacturing process for creating the UpCircle Shampoo Crème is too complex to recreate at home due to its hybrid solid/liquid consistency. Instead, here I'm sharing a simple solid bar recipe to suit as many hair types as possible. Switching shampoo, especially if you've been using a traditional liquid shampoo, will mean that your hair needs time to adjust. There might be a build-up from other products in your hair, so adapting to something new can take several weeks. Feel free to experiment with other oils or waxes if it needs tweaking for your specific hair's needs.

01 Start by following the instructions on page 133 to make your homemade ginger oil.

02 Fill the saucepan with about 5 cm (2 in) water and bring to a simmer over medium heat. Place the heatproof bowl on top of the saucepan, ensuring it fits securely without touching the water. Add the carnuba wax and allow to melt, stirring occasionally.

03 Once melted, let it cool slightly and then add all other ingredients. Stir thoroughly.

04 Pour the mixture into your mould, then let it set in the fridge for at least 4 hours or overnight. Your shampoo bar should last 5–6 months, but with regular hair washing you may have used it up in less time.

05 To use, first wet your hair thoroughly. Some people like to apply the bar directly to the hair and scalp, my preference is to build the lather by rubbing it into my wet hands. Work the product into your hair, focusing on the scalp and roots. Rinse your hair thoroughly with warm water until all the shampoo is washed out.

THE WHY:

• Ginger oil is great for boosting the circulation in your scalp, and this in turn can help to minimise dryness and flaking. It also has a similar reputation as rosemary oil for stimulating hair growth and strengthening the hair. In addition, apple cider vinegar helps to balance the pH of your scalp and boost shine.

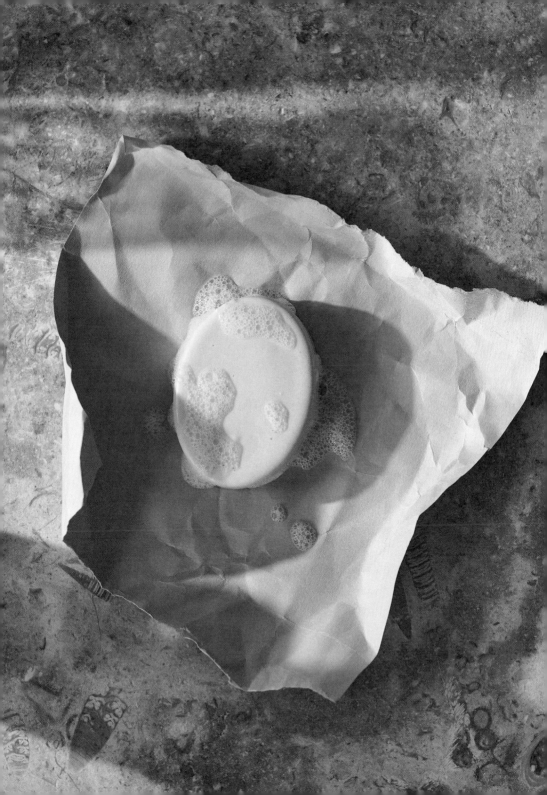

SCRUBS

When we launched UpCircle, scrubs were our very first product and they remain to this day the signature of our range. For that reason, I'll always be a big advocate of a hardworking, gentle scrub for both the face and body.

Many things came together at the same time to push my brother and I to make the decision of risking it all to start UpCircle. One of those things was the microbead scandal. This was the horrendous realisation that the vast majority of face scrubs, washes and toothpastes contained thousands of these tiny plastic beads which, once flushed down our sinks or showers, could never ever be filtered back out of the water supply.

So, what could we use to replace these tiny terrors? There are SO many options. The best thing about all the natural, biodegradable alternatives available is that most have their own specific skincare benefits too. Plus, of course, many of them can be found in your kitchen cabinets.

If you have leftovers of any of these scrubs, store the remainder in a reusable, air-tight container and use within 3 days (but much better used immediately!).

COFFEE BODY SCRUB

**MAKES APPROX.
150 G (5 OZ)** – *one large jar*

INGREDIENTS:

about 100 g *(3½ oz)* fresh coffee
grounds
10 g *(¼ oz)* fine sea salt
20 g *(¾ oz)* fine sugar *(I tend to use
brown, cane or rapadura)*
2 tablespoons coconut oil
2 tablespoons almond oil *(olive or
avocado oil also work)*
4–5 drops of the essential oil of
your choice *(see tip)*

YOU WILL NEED:

glass jar with a lid

TIP:

*If you want to recreate the
UpCircle Body Scrub it is made
with lemongrass and lime
essential oils. Another gorgeous
combo is to combine peppermint
and eucalyptus essential oils –
use a couple of drops of each.*

I've hosted 'make your own scrub' events in cafés, at conferences, in offices, at markets, in uni halls – you name it! They're a lot of fun and the process is incredibly simple, so it's an easy one to do regularly at home. It'll come as no surprise that I've picked coffee as the key ingredient here. Coffee is what started UpCircle, and we collect over 100 kg (220 lb) of this gorgeous ingredient every day. We collect the grounds from cafés and restaurants and use them to make tens of thousands of scrubs per year.

This recipe is almost exactly the same as our infamous body scrub, the product that we are best-known for. First and foremost, I wouldn't advise making too much at once. Make a fresh coffee, either with a cafetière or using a machine that produces coffee grounds, and use only what you've made from that one day. This is the exact approach we take to our large scale coffee collections. They take place every day and we only collect coffee grounds that have been produced in that one given day – it's never stored or collected over time. Let's get started!

01 Measure all the ingredients into a medium bowl and stir to combine. If you've made enough to store for more than one use, transfer to a jar with a lid and store in the fridge for up to 3 days.

02 To use, apply in the bath or shower onto damp skin. Massage the scrub into the skin in circular motions. For the full effect, leave on the skin for 3–5 minutes before washing off.

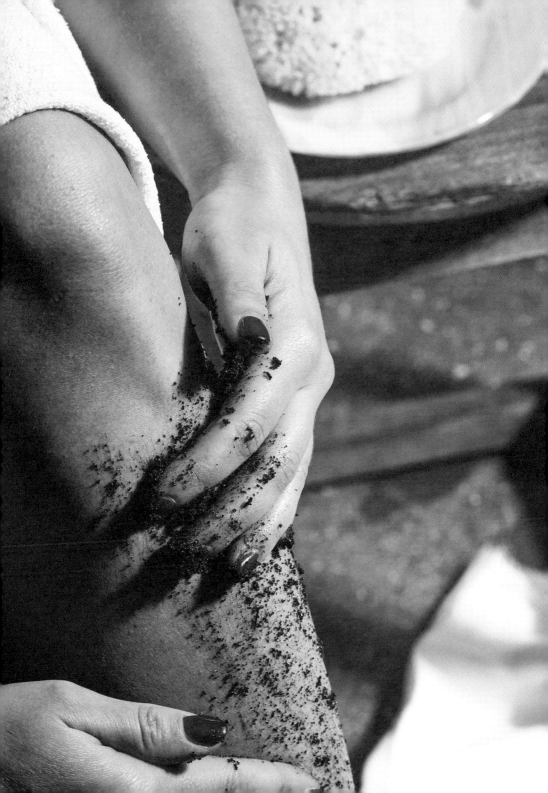

COFFEE FACE SCRUB

INGREDIENTS:

about 100 g *(3½ oz)* fresh coffee
    grounds
10 g *(¼ oz)* fine sea salt *(optional)*
2 tablespoons coconut oil
2 tablespoons almond oil *(olive or
    avocado oil also work)*
2–3 drops of the essential oil of
    your choice *(see below)*

FOR SENSITIVE SKIN:

rose
rosehip
chamomile
patchouli
lavender
jasmine
ylang–ylang

FOR DRY OR DEHYDRATED SKIN:

lemon verbena
sweet orange
bergamot
apricot
grapefruit

FOR OILY, CONGESTED
OR SPOT-PRONE SKIN:

tea tree
petitgrain
rosemary
thyme
peppermint

The process for this is almost identical to that for the body scrub on page 44, with just a few minor tweaks. The skin on your face is more delicate, so it's vital to ensure your face scrub won't cause micro tears or irritate your skin. It's important to ensure that the texture is super soft, that you carefully select your essential oils based on your skin type, and that your skin is wet on application. Scrub with less vigour than you would on your thighs!

01 Let's focus on texture first. For the face, we remove the sugar from the body scrub recipe. If you'd still like to use salt (fantastic for combating breakouts), make sure it's very fine. You can use just coffee for the face scrub – as an exfoliant, it is much softer than sugar or salt, and should be suitable for all skin types.

02 Next, the essential oils. It's important to choose oils that work with your skin type. See ingredients.

03 Go easy on the essential oils – a couple of drops should be sufficient. And if you're not sure? My top pick, regardless of skin type, has to be rosehip oil!

04 And lastly, make sure your skin is wet before you apply the face scrub. Applying the scrub to a dry face will increase the risk of irritation.

05 If you have any left over, store in an air-tight reusable container in the fridge for up to 3 days.

THE WHY:

- You just need to try this once to understand the 'why'! The scents are absolutely beautiful and this scrub leaves your skin feeling incredibly soft, smooth and moisturised. The fine coffee grounds act as a natural exfoliator, helping to buff away dry and dead skin, while the caffeine in the coffee helps stimulate blood flow, making it effective against skin conditions such as acne, eczema and cellulite (when used on the body). It helps to address areas in need of renewal and regeneration. Coffee is the same pH as your skin, meaning it won't leave it feeling dry. The oils in this recipe also leave your skin with a beautiful glowy, healthy look. What's not to love?

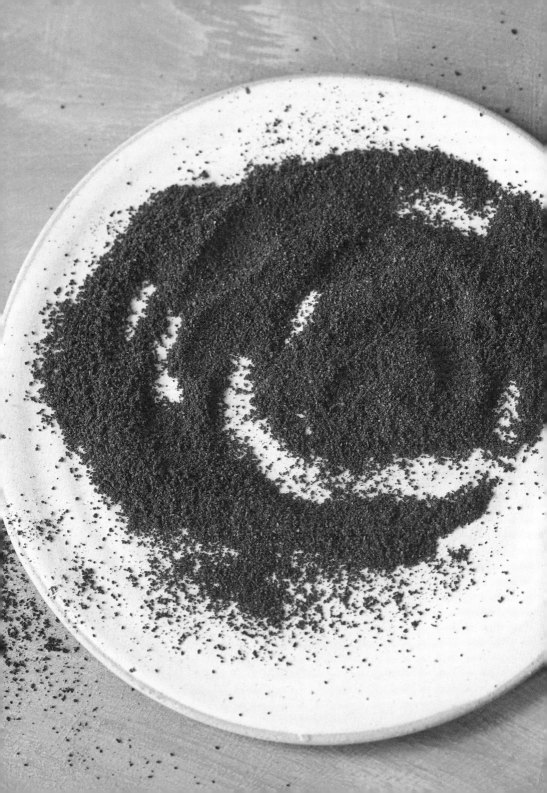

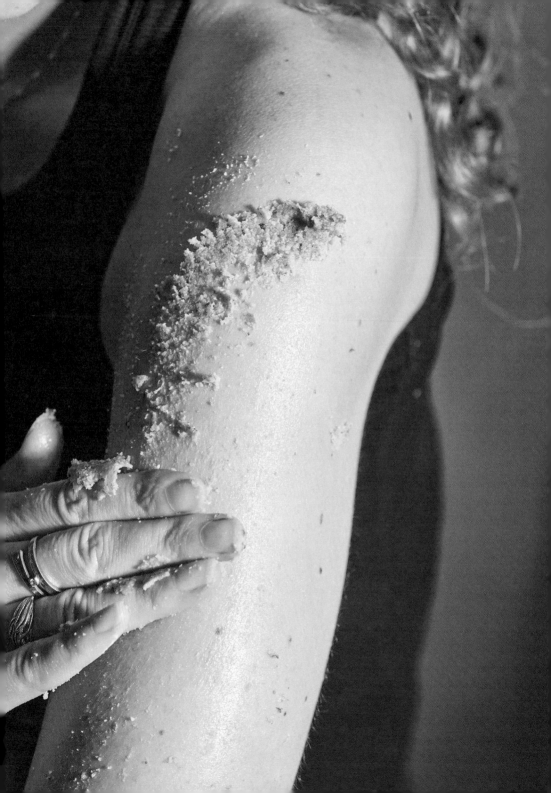

SWEET OAT + LIME BODY SCRUB

MAKES 3 TREATMENTS

INGREDIENTS:

8 tablespoons rolled oats
peel of 1–2 limes
2 tablespoons brown sugar
2 tablespoons coconut oil

YOU WILL NEED:

heatproof bowl and saucepan
  to create a bain-marie/
  double-boiler
glass jar with a lid

TIP:

Coffee grounds can go down the drain no problem, but if you have any worries about this oat scrub, place a drain saver (I use a small piece of an old mesh strainer) over the plughole to catch any of the larger bits.

This is a scrub to feed and replenish the uppermost layers of skin. I love it because it includes only four ingredients, all of which you probably have in your kitchen cabinets already. Oats are a real superhero ingredient as they contain natural ceramides that can soothe inflamed and irritated skin. If you're not a coffee fan, oats are a great alternative for a scrub.

01 Add the oats to a food processor and pulse until finely ground. Next, add the peel and pulse a little more. Transfer to a bowl and add the sugar, and mix together.

02 Fill the saucepan with about 5 cm (2 in) water and bring to a simmer over a medium heat. Place the heatproof bowl on top of the saucepan, ensuring it fits securely without touching the water. Add the coconut oil to the bowl and stir occasionally until fully melted.

03 Pour the melted coconut oil into the bowl with the other ingredients and stir thoroughly. If the consistency is too dry, you can add another tablespoon of coconut oil. Transfer to a jar with a lid and store in the fridge for up to 7 days.

04 To use, apply the scrub to damp skin in the bath or shower. Massage the scrub into the skin in circular motions. For the full effect, leave on the skin for 3–5 minutes before washing off.

THE WHY:

- Oats are full of antioxidants and anti-inflammatory compounds known for moisturising dry skin and providing relief from itching, rashes and other minor skin irritations. Lime peel contains citric acid, which has natural exfoliating properties. It's also an excellent source of vitamin C, a potent antioxidant that helps neutralise free radicals and protect the skin from oxidative stress. Vitamin C is also crucial for collagen synthesis, which is essential for maintaining skin elasticity and firmness. The lime peel also makes this scrub smell diviiiiine!

OAT + CARROT
FACE SCRUB

MAKES 3 SCRUBS

INGREDIENTS:

2 tablespoons rolled oats
1 carrot, grated
2 teaspoons coconut oil
1 teaspoon almond oil

YOU WILL NEED:

heatproof bowl and saucepan
to create a bain-marie/
double-boiler
glass jar with a lid

This scrub is mainly carrot with added ground oats, rather than the other way around. Just like with your coffee face scrub, the oats in this recipe must be very finely ground to be suitable for use on the face. Allow more time in the blender to accommodate.

01 Tip the oats into a blender and blitz until very finely ground. Transfer into a bowl and add the grated carrot.

02 Fill the saucepan with about 5 cm (2 in) water and bring to a simmer over a medium heat. Place the heatproof bowl on top of the saucepan, ensuring it fits securely without touching the water. Add the coconut oil to the bowl and stir occasionally until fully melted.

03 Add the melted coconut oil to the bowl with the carrots and oats, along with the almond oil. Mix well to combine. Transfer to a jar with a lid and store in the fridge for up to 7 days.

04 To use, wet your face and neck before applying the scrub to your entire face with your fingertips. Massage in gently, then let sit for 4–6 minutes. Rinse off with a washcloth and warm water.

THE WHY:

- Carrots are well known for their high content of beta-carotene, a powerful antioxidant that helps protect the skin from free-radical damage caused by environmental stressors like UV rays and pollution. It also contributes to skin-cell renewal and repair, promoting a healthy complexion.

SWEET GRAPEFRUIT LIP SCRUB

MAKES 4 TREATMENTS

INGREDIENTS:

1 teaspoon coconut oil
approx. 3 teaspoons finely grated
   grapefruit peel
½ teaspoon fine brown sugar

YOU WILL NEED:

heatproof bowl and saucepan
   to create a bain-marie
   /double-boiler
small glass jar, about the size of
   a typical lip balm container,
   with a lid

Grapefruit is one of my favourite fruits. I hated it as a child, but I have done a complete 180 as an adult. Home-squeezed grapefruit juice is just unbeatable in my opinion, but of course it leaves you with copious amounts of peels. The good news is, they contain a whole lotta goodness! If you're not a fan of grapefruit, orange peel (or indeed any other citrus peel) also works well here.

01 Fill the saucepan with about 5 cm (2 in) water and bring to a simmer over a medium heat. Place the heatproof bowl on top of the saucepan, ensuring it fits securely without touching the water. Add the coconut oil to the bowl and stir occasionally until fully melted. Remove from the heat and stir in the grated grapefruit peel, then set aside to cool slightly.

02 When the mixture is tepid, add the sugar. If it's too hot, the sugar will dissolve and you want a bit of grittiness. Scoop the mixture into a jar with a lid and store in the fridge for up to 5 days.

03 To use, gently rub the scrub into your lips! They should be left feeling softer and smoother, and the flavour of the scrub should linger slightly too – delicious!

SEE IMAGE OVERLEAF

THE WHY:

- Like lemons and all citrus, grapefruit has natural acids that help to exfoliate dead skin. The vitamin C in the peel helps boost hydration and moisture retention, keeping your lips supple and chap-free.

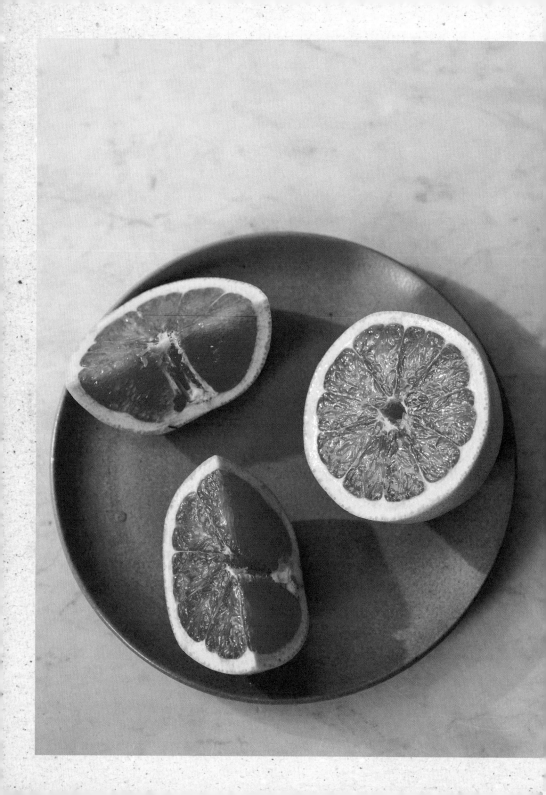

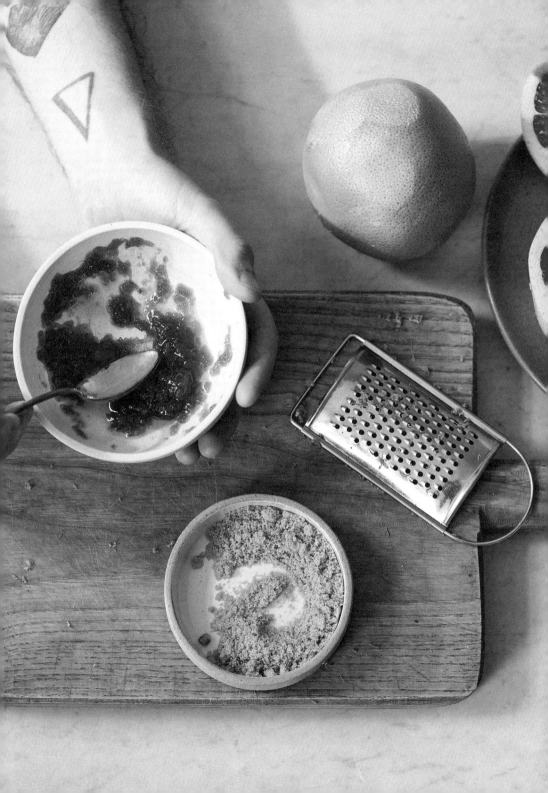

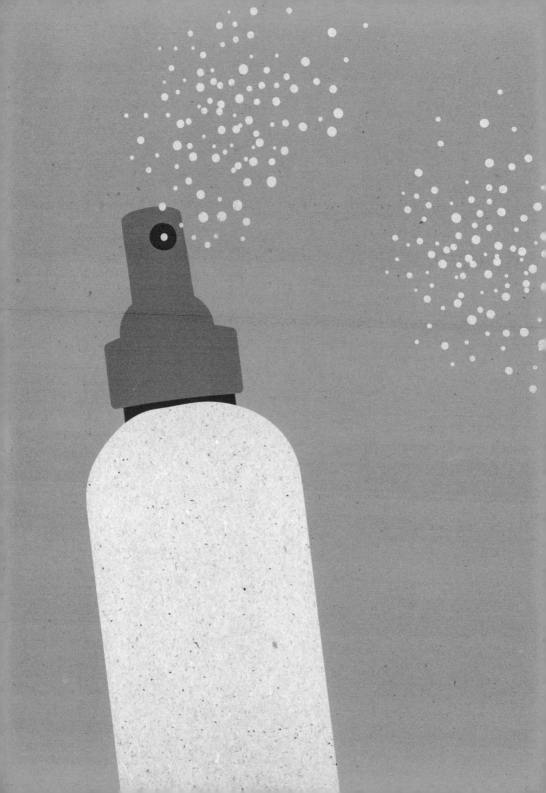

OILS + MISTS

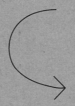

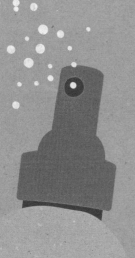

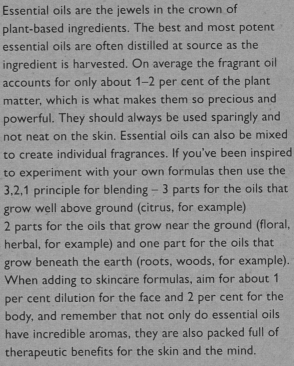

Essential oils are the jewels in the crown of plant-based ingredients. The best and most potent essential oils are often distilled at source as the ingredient is harvested. On average the fragrant oil accounts for only about 1–2 per cent of the plant matter, which is what makes them so precious and powerful. They should always be used sparingly and not neat on the skin. Essential oils can also be mixed to create individual fragrances. If you've been inspired to experiment with your own formulas then use the 3,2,1 principle for blending – 3 parts for the oils that grow well above ground (citrus, for example) 2 parts for the oils that grow near the ground (floral, herbal, for example) and one part for the oils that grow beneath the earth (roots, woods, for example). When adding to skincare formulas, aim for about 1 per cent dilution for the face and 2 per cent for the body, and remember that not only do essential oils have incredible aromas, they are also packed full of therapeutic benefits for the skin and the mind.

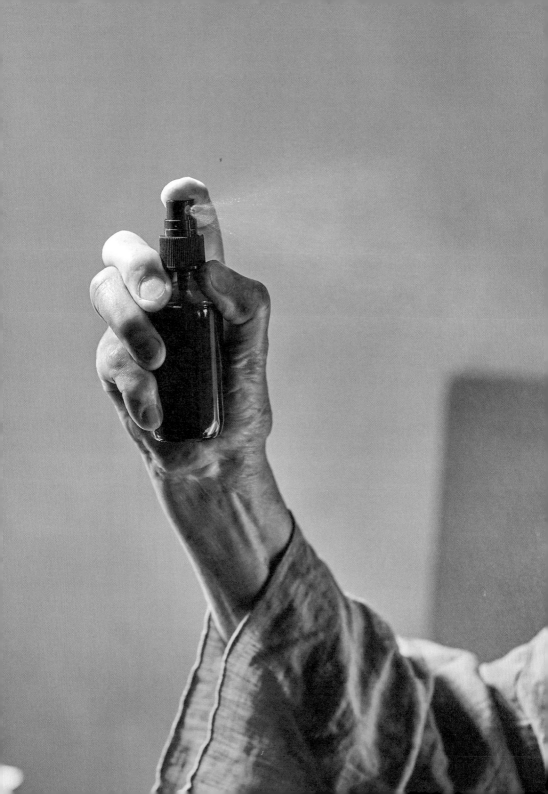

A NOTE ON ESSENTIAL OILS

As you might have guessed from the chapter intro, some of the recipes in this section use essential oils or homemade infused oils (see pages 131–139). Essential oils normally last about two years if kept in a cool, dark place and you only need a few drops, so they are very cost-effective. If you know you'll be using your essential oils very irregularly, pop them in the fridge to keep them fresher for longer.

Prioritise expensive oils like rose and jasmine for leave-on skincare products, like serums and moisturisers, and use less-expensive oils for things like bath oils.

Add the oils drop by drop, and don't be tempted to add more. A little essential oil can soothe the mind, body and soul, but too much can give you a headache or irritate your skin. Stronger-smelling oils include eucalyptus, peppermint, bay, basil, lime, lemon, thyme and rosemary, so be aware of this when adding them to your products.

Essential oils can have a significant effect not just on your body but on your mind. Here's a little chart for how you can pair your choice of oils with how you're feeling. I've given suggested quantities for adding to a bath, so adjust as necessary if you're using them in other ways.

BERGAMOT ESSENTIAL OIL	for balancing or improving your mood	5 DROPS
CHAMOMILE ESSENTIAL OIL	for insomnia or itchy skin	7 DROPS
FRANKINCENSE ESSENTIAL OIL	for calming and mood-sweetening	8 DROPS
GERANIUM ESSENTIAL OIL	for relaxing yet uplifting and energising	10 DROPS
YLANG-YLANG ESSENTIAL OIL	for boredom, stress or fatigue	8 DROPS
LAVENDER ESSENTIAL OIL	for boosting positivity, soothing and relaxing	10 DROPS
NEROLI ESSENTIAL OIL	for relieving stress and anxiety	8 DROPS

PLUMPING CINNAMON LIP OIL

INGREDIENTS:

7-8 drops of Cinnamon Oil *(see page 137)*
½ teaspoon coconut oil, melted
½ teaspoon almond oil

YOU WILL NEED:

small rollerball bottle or small bottle with a pipette

TIP:

When applied topically, cinnamon usually causes a tingling sensation. This is normal and part of the plumping effect. However, if you experience any irritation or discomfort, discontinue use.

I whip up a homemade cinnamon oil every January. I make myself a festive wreath every November and it always has cinnamon sticks in it. The thought of using them only for a decoration does not sit well with me, so, of course, I have to find a way to give the cinnamon a second life in one way or another.

01 Start by making the homemade cinnamon oil on page 137.

02 Mix the ingredients together in a small bowl and then carefully transfer to your chosen bottle. I use a rollerball bottle for lip oil as it prevents me from using too much on each application, but you can also use a small bottle with a pipette dropper and just drop a single drop onto your fingertip to apply.

03 To use, apply directly to clean, dry lips.

04 The oil will keep for up to 6 months if stored appropriately, away from heat and direct sunlight.

THE WHY:

- That tingling sensation described above is due to increasing blood flow, and causes the lips to appear fuller and more voluminous. Additionally, cinnamon oil possesses antioxidant properties that help protect the delicate skin of the lips from environmental damage and premature ageing. The choice of avocado oil as a carrier in this instance was not accidental. Avocado oil is brilliant for lips, as it's a great source of vitamin E. It's also rich in oleic acid, which helps to lock in moisture and prevent dryness. It penetrates deeply into the skin, leaving your lips soft, smooth and supple. The antioxidants and vitamins in avocado oil also help to repair damaged lips.

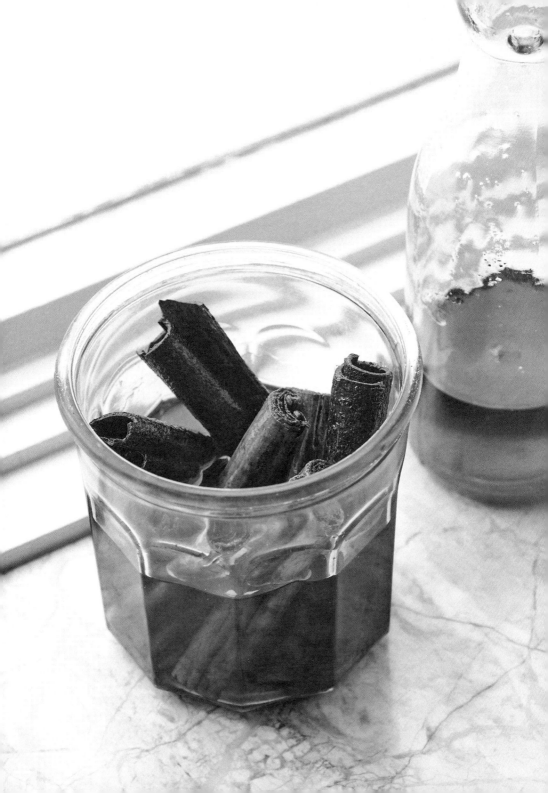

AVOCADO CUTICLE OIL

**MAKES ABOUT 50 ML
(2 FL OZ)**

INGREDIENTS:

skins and stones of 3–5 avocados
carrier oil of your choice, such as
   olive oil, almond oil or
   grapeseed oil

YOU WILL NEED:

glass jar, about the size of a large
   jam jar
saucepan
fine-mesh strainer or piece of
   muslin *(cheesecloth)*
small rollerball bottle or small
   bottle with a pipette

TIP:

*Generally, what's good for
your nails is also good for your
hair. This doubles up as a hair
oil; when you get out of the
shower, apply a few drops to
your fingertips and massage
into the ends of clean, damp
hair. It's great for preventing
breakages and split ends.*

Here, we use avocado stones and skin to make an oil for conditioning and promoting strong, healthy nails – so if you've made a batch of guac, this is an ideal way to use them up! Avocado oil is great for softening cuticles and strengthening nails, so I use pure avocado oil on mine whenever I remove varnish, to help restore and rehydrate them. Our head of content Giulia gave me this tip. Her hands often feature on our social media and her nails are so strong that we get frequent comments from people assuming she's wearing long plastic nails. In fact, they are completely natural, very well-looked-after nails – all thanks to avocado!

01 Allow the avocado stones and skins to air-dry for a couple of days before starting the process of making your oil.

02 When you're ready, peel the outer layer of your avocado stones using a knife or sharp peeler. This should flake off super easily as the outer layer usually separates from the inner layer of the stone as they dry out.

03 Cut the stones into cubes; this increases the surface area and allows for more infusion into the oil. For the same reason, tear your skins into smaller pieces.

04 Transfer the stones and skins into your jar and pour over enough carrier oil to cover.

05 Pour water into the saucepan to a depth of about 7.5 cm (3 in) and bring to the boil over a medium heat. Place your jar (lid off!!) into the water and leave to simmer for 10 minutes.

06 Remove the pan from the heat, but keep the jar in the pan overnight. In the morning, strain your oil to remove the stones and skins. It should look slightly greener than extra virgin olive oil. Transfer the oil into your chosen storage bottle. The oil will keep for 6 months if stored appropriately, away from heat and direct sunlight.

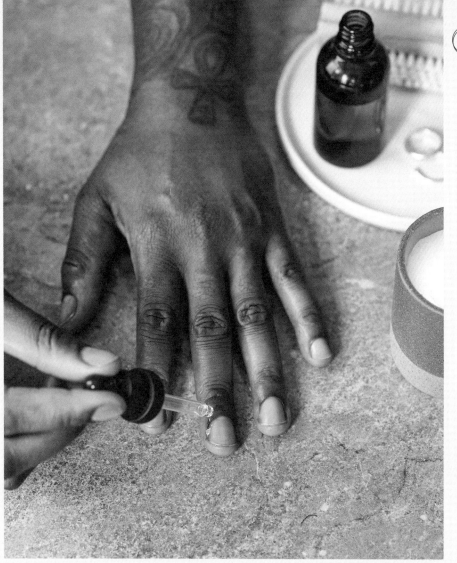

07 To use, first wash and thoroughly dry your hands. Add a single drop to each nail bed and massage in. This is particularly good when used after removing varnish or a manicure/pedicure. (Works for toes, too!)

THE WHY:

- Avocado contains potassium, which promotes keratin production. This can prevent your nails from becoming brittle, while also encouraging growth.

HAIR OIL
with browning or wilted herbs

MAKES APPROX. 100 ML (3½ FL OZ)

Revive and nourish your hair with this oil that promotes healthy hair growth and adds shine.

INGREDIENTS:

8 tablespoons of your favourite carrier oil such as coconut oil, jojoba oil or almond oil *(see tip)*
handful of wilted herbs, such as rosemary, basil, mint or thyme

YOU WILL NEED:

reusable glass jar with a secure lid
saucepan *(optional)*
fine-mesh strainer or a piece of muslin *(cheesecloth)*
glass bottle with a secure lid or pipette

TIP:

Choose a carrier oil suitable for your hair type and preferences. Coconut oil is deeply nourishing, jojoba oil closely resembles the natural sebum of your scalp, and almond oil is lightweight and moisturising.

01 Pour your chosen carrier oil into your clean glass jar. Add the wilted herbs, ensuring the herbs are completely submerged in the oil. Close the jar with a secure lid.

02 If you have some time and want to maximise the herb infusion, place the sealed jar near a sunny window for a week. Sunlight can help extract more herbal properties into the oil.

03 However, if you prefer a faster infusion, you can use the stove method. Place the sealed jar in a saucepan filled with water over a low heat. Leave on the heat for 1–2 hours, ensuring the oil doesn't overheat. This gentle heating process helps the herbs release their beneficial properties into the oil. Let the oil cool to room temperature.

04 After the infusion process (whether you've used the sun or stove method), strain the infused oil into a clean bowl, discarding the wilted herbs. Transfer the herb-infused hair oil into a clean glass bottle with a secure lid. The oil will keep for 6 months if stored appropriately, away from heat and direct sunlight.

05 To use, apply a small amount of the herb-infused hair oil to your scalp and hair, massaging it gently. Leave it on for at least 30 minutes or overnight for deeper conditioning. Shampoo and condition your hair as usual to reveal nourished and revitalised locks!

THE WHY:

- The combination of herbs and plant-based oil here helps nourish and condition your hair, making it softer and more manageable. The infusion of herbs imparts a natural shine, leaving your hair looking lustrous and radiant. Rosemary helps to support hair growth and stimulate the scalp, encouraging healthier and stronger hair.

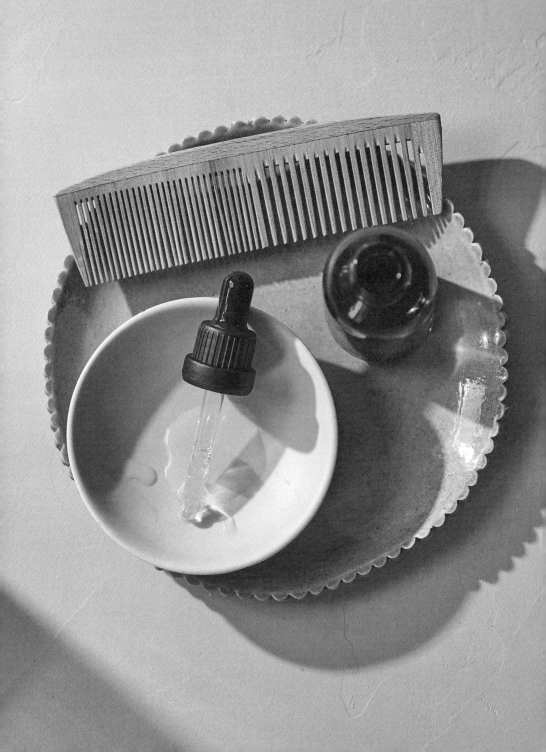

EYEBROW *or* EYELASH OIL

**MAKES ENOUGH FOR
2 TREATMENTS**

INGREDIENTS:

2–3 drops of the herb infusion you
created for your hair oil
(see page 62)
4–5 drops of castor oil

YOU WILL NEED:

small dish for mixing
glass bottle with secure lid or pipette
cotton bud or brow brush (optional)

The infused herbal oil on the previous page can also be used to make an eyebrow or eyelash oil for brows and lashes that appear healthy and well looked after. It also helps with grooming them into your desired shape/direction.

01 Mix the ingredients together in a small dish.

02 Transfer the herb-infused oil into a clean glass bottle with a secure lid. The oil will keep for 6 months if stored appropriately, away from heat and direct sunlight.

03 Use either your fingertips or a cotton bud or a clean mascara wand / brow brush to apply to clean, dry brows or lashes.

TIP:

To nourish your eyelashes, put a tiny bit of pure castor oil onto the end of your clean, dry fingertip and slowly blink your lashes onto your finger. Repeat a couple of times per eye. If you'd rather, you can apply with a cotton bud (bamboo sticks only, please!) or clean mascara wand. With daily application, you should see results in about 30 days, with thicker, longer lashes.

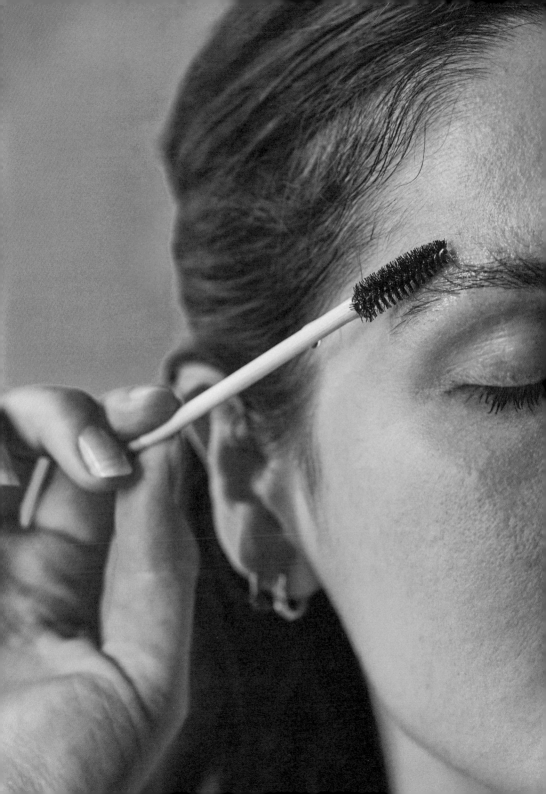

ORANGE PEEL BODY OIL

**MAKES APPROX. 150 ML
(5 FL OZ)**

INGREDIENTS:

8 tablespoons grapeseed oil
 (or any carrier oil of your choice)
1 tablespoon jojoba oil
1 tablespoon Apricot Kernel Oil
 (see page 136)
10 drops of your Orange Peel Oil
 (see page 135)
5 drops of Lemon Peel Oil
 (see page 134)
3 drops of bergamot essential oil

YOU WILL NEED:

tinted 150 ml (5 fl oz) glass
 container with a lid

TIP:

It's preferable to use a dark or amber-coloured glass bottle to protect the oils from sunlight, which can cause them to degrade over time.

The main things I'm looking for in a body oil are that it makes my skin look healthy, nourished and scale-free. I also want it to smell great – this one has a fruity, fresh summery scent that I LOVE. Here, we use homemade apricot kernel oil as well as orange and lemon peel oils in the body oil for citrusy goodness.

01 Start by following the instructions on pages 134–136 to make your homemade citrus peel oils and apricot kernel oil.

02 In a small bowl, combine the grapeseed oil, jojoba oil and apricot kernel oil. Now carefully add the orange, lemon and bergamot oils to the carrier oil mixture. Stir the mixture gently to ensure the essential oils are well distributed. Carefully pour the fruity oil into the glass container. Seal the container with the lid tightly. The oil will keep for 6 months if stored appropriately, away from heat and direct sunlight.

03 To use, apply a small amount of the body oil onto your skin after a bath or shower. Gently massage the oil into your skin in circular motions, allowing it to absorb fully. Enjoy the fruity aroma and the moisturising benefits of the body oil. It will leave your skin feeling soft, smooth and nourished.

THE WHY:

• The carrier oils used here (grapeseed, jojoba and apricot kernel) are light and non-greasy, and they absorb well into the skin, making them ideal for use in a body oil. The citrus oils not only provide a refreshing fruity aroma, but also offer mood-lifting and skin-brightening properties.

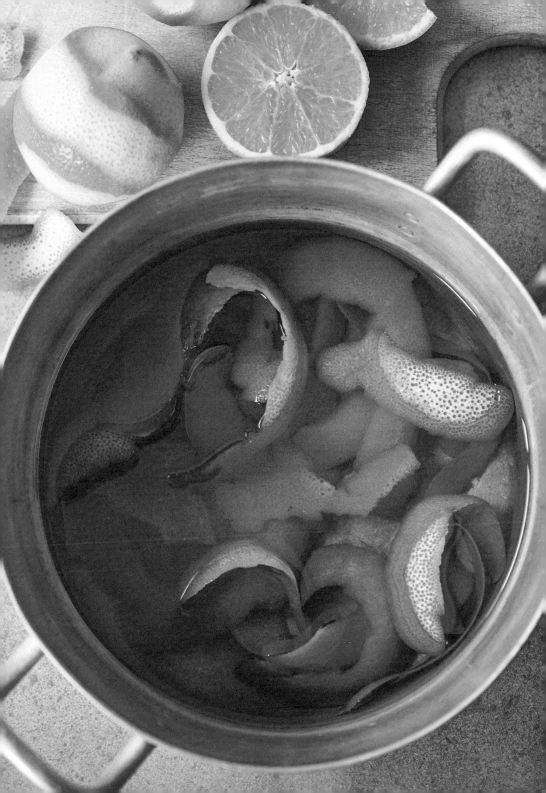

ROSE WATER
FACE MIST

MAKES 250 ML (8½ FL OZ)

INGREDIENTS:

250 ml *(8½ fl oz)* distilled or
  filtered water
as many sad-looking rose petals
  as you have – ideally at least
  5 roses' worth
1 teaspoon vegetable glycerine
  (optional)

YOU WILL NEED:

saucepan
fine-mesh strainer
reusable glass spray bottle

> **TIP:**
> *Store your mist in the fridge for
> an extra-refreshing spritz!*

With this recipe, you can create your own rose water using 'past their best' roses that you've had on display. I'm always rescuing bouquets from tables at events and bringing them home for a longer life – in the end, they become bath salts (see page 96) and drawer fresheners (see page 106) or face mists, like this one!

01 Pour the distilled or filtered water into the saucepan and bring to a gentle boil over a medium heat. Once it reaches the boil, turn off the heat and add the rose petals to the water. Leave to steep for about 20–30 minutes.

02 After the steeping time, strain the rose-petal infusion through a fine-mesh strainer into a clean bowl. Squeeze the petals to extract as much liquid as possible, then discard (the petals can be composted).

03 Add the glycerine to the infusion, if desired. Vegetable glycerine acts as a humectant, attracting moisture to your skin and enhancing the mist's hydrating properties. If you prefer a simpler mist, you can omit this step.

04 Carefully pour the rose-petal face mist into a reusable glass spray bottle. This will keep for a month in the fridge.

05 To use, hold the nozzle 20–30 cm (8–12 in) from clean, dry or slightly damp face and spritz 3 or 4 times. Wait for it to dry before applying any other products.

THE WHY:

- Rose petals are rich in natural oils and water, providing your skin with much-needed hydration and a refreshing boost. They also contain antioxidants that help promote skin's radiance and combat early signs of ageing. This face mist is gentle and suitable for all skin types, including sensitive skin.

SEA SALT HAIR-TEXTURISING MIST

MAKES ABOUT 230 ML (8 FL OZ)

INGREDIENTS:

225 ml *(8 fl oz)* warm water
about 1 tablespoon leftover salt
1 teaspoon coconut oil
2–3 drops of your fave essential
  oil *(I'd recommend rosemary
  or coconut, or, if you're wanting
  to enhance the lime, then lime,
  lemon verbena or lemongrass)*

YOU WILL NEED:

spritzing bottle *(such as an old
  toner spray bottle)*

When I see salt sprays and mists on the shelves in shops, I really don't understand it, because they are so unbelievably easy to make at home. I tend to make a fresh batch of this spray whenever I've hosted a drinks party and ended up making cocktails with a salt rim. To make the salt rims, I usually have a plate of lime juice to pop the glass into first, then I pour out my lovely sea salt flakes onto a second plate and dip the glass into them next. Of course, there is always limey salt left over that I don't want to throw away – so then it's texture mist-making time!

01 Mix all the ingredients together in a jug until well combined, then decant into the bottle. The mist will keep for 6 months if stored appropriately, away from heat and direct sunlight.

02 To apply, hold the nozzle 20–30 cm (8–12 in) from clean, dry or slightly damp hair, and spritz generously. The more you spritz, the more textured your hair will be, but be careful – go too far, and your hair will start to feel crunchy or look powdery. I have long, slightly wavy but thick hair, and usually use up to 10 spritzes.

THE WHY:

- This works brilliantly if you're trying to make an updo keep its shape a little more easily. If you have fine, slippery hair that never stays put, then this could be a game-changer for you.

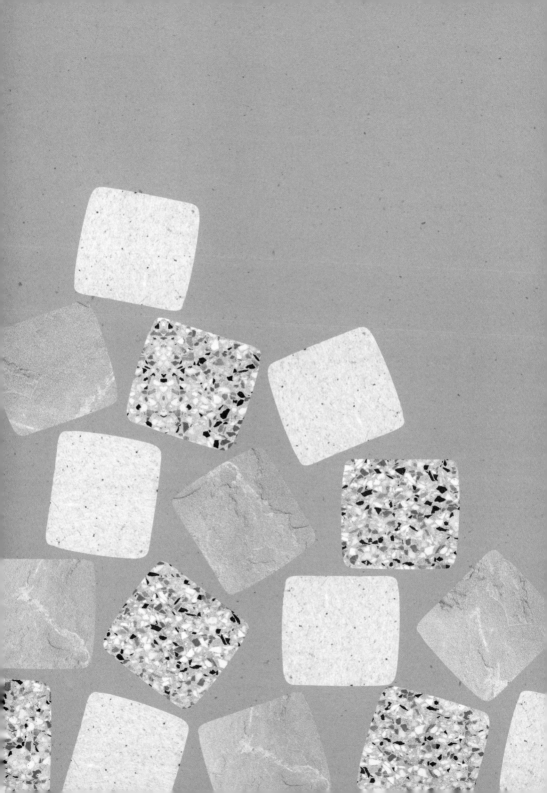

ICES

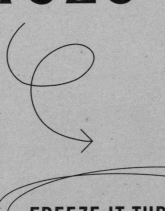

FREEZE IT THREE WAYS!

What I love about frozen skincare treats is that you don't have to worry about using them within a particular timeframe. So if you've got fresh ingredients that are 'on the turn', converting them into a frozen skin or scalp treatment is a great way to avoid them ending up in the bin.

Cooling treatments also hold a plethora of benefits – in the hot summer months, I keep most of my daily skincare in the fridge simply because it's refreshing. But cold skincare can also help to minimise the appearance of large pores, as well as reduce redness, swelling and puffiness.

Here are three frozen treatments that I keep in a Tupperware in my freezer!

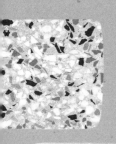

COLD COFFEE FACIAL

**MAKES ENOUGH
FOR 2–3 FACIALS**

INGREDIENTS:

leftover black coffee

YOU WILL NEED:

ice-cube tray
soft piece of muslin *(cheesecloth)*

The scrubs chapter provides recipes that make use of coffee grounds, but what about coffee water left behind in your cafetiere? Don't worry, there's a use for that too! How much this makes depends on how much coffee you have to use up.

01 Pour your leftover coffee into the ice-cube tray and freeze until solid.

02 To use, take a cube (or you could use a few) and wrap in the muslin cloth. I like to wait a couple of minutes for it to soften slightly and for the cube(s) to begin slightly melting through the cloth. When you're ready, massage gently into your face in circular motions. If you want to rinse your face after, you can, but this is not essential.

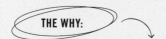

THE WHY:

- This treatment temporarily reduces swelling and puffiness. The caffeine is high in antioxidants and increases blood circulation, leading to brighter, fresher-looking skin. In addition, any facial is a calming act of self-care, which is great for stress and anxiety.

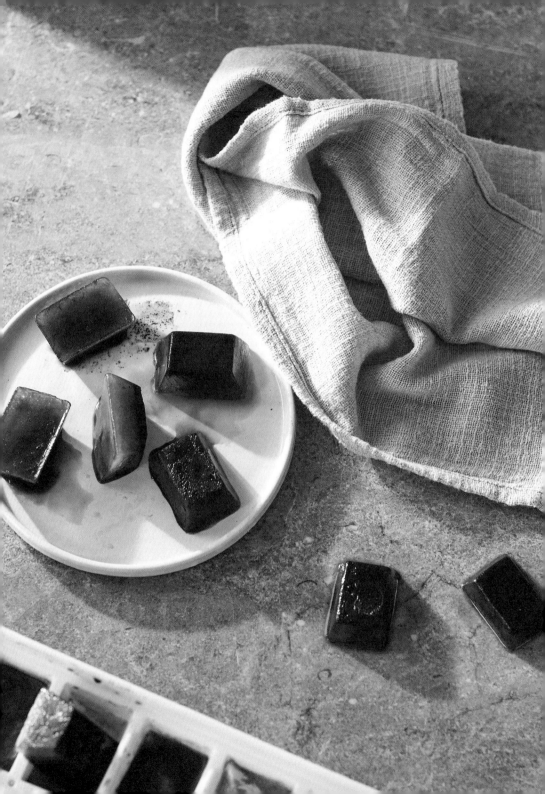

ROSEMARY-INFUSED SCALP MASSAGER

MAKES 2 MASSAGE BARS

INGREDIENTS:

handful of browning rosemary
handful of wilting mint
400–500 ml *(13–17 fl oz)* water

YOU WILL NEED:

saucepan
fine-mesh strainer
silicone massager mould *(see tip)*

> **TIP:**
>
> *The silicone massager moulds can also be used for body butter bars, soaps and solid scrub bars – even bath bombs! The bobbles make the bar less slippery in your hand than a traditional mould, and are less likely to get stuck to the edge of your sink or bath once wet.*

Scalp care is the first step in haircare and should never be overlooked on the journey to healthy hair. Think of this cooling massager as a scalp facial! Silicone massager moulds are very inexpensive and widely available, so if you're looking for just one style of mould, this is what I would opt for – if not, large silicone ice cube moulds also do the job!

01 Combine the rosemary, mint and water in a small saucepan over a medium heat. Bring to the boil and simmer for 10 minutes.

02 Strain the water into a bowl to remove the sprigs and leaves. Leave to cool, then pour into your moulds and freeze.

03 To use, remove a bar from the mould and brush through wet hair before focusing on massaging it into the scalp in circular motions. Take your time and make slow but firm movements. Continue your usual haircare routine after use.

THE WHY:

• There is evidence that rosemary not only prevents hair loss but also stimulates new hair growth. Additionally, it defends against free radicals and offers protection against UV damage. The act of massaging something solid into your scalp also helps to cleanse, hydrate and 'wake up' your scalp by exfoliating dead skin and encouraging blood flow.

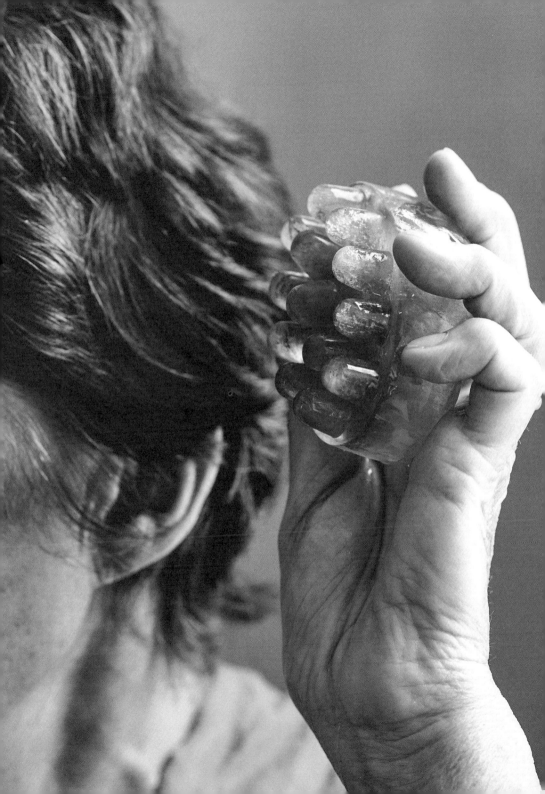

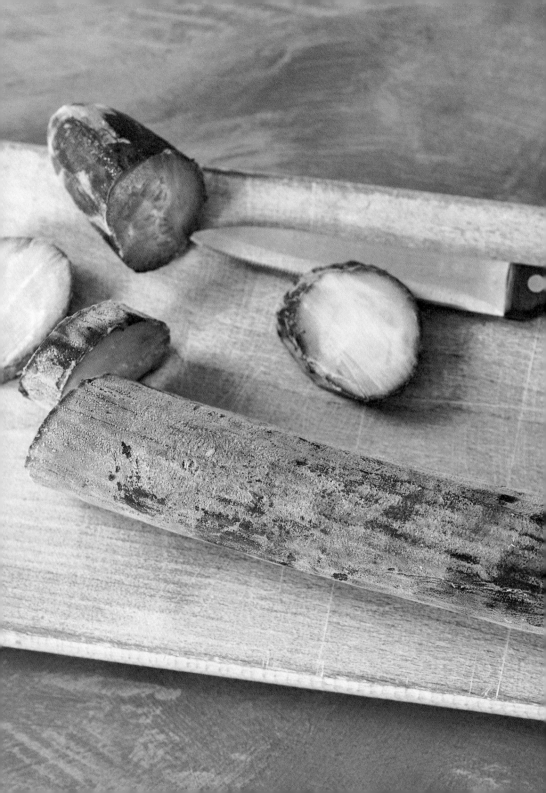

CUCUMBER FACIAL

INGREDIENTS:

1 cucumber *(or a part-used one!)*

I am definitely guilty of buying a cucumber almost solely for use as G&T garnish. By the Thursday following my weekend, I worry that I won't be able to use it up in time... That's why there's usually a part-used cucumber in my freezer! Luckily, it's the perfect way to give yourself a cooling facial. I do this in the morning for glowy, soft skin that has that lovely dewy look.

01 Place your cucumber into the freezer. Make sure it is stored somewhere clean – pop it in a Tupperware if needs be. Freeze!

02 To use, cleanse your skin as normal, then slice the very end of the cucumber so you have a clean surface. Glide the cut end of the cucumber slowly across your skin. Take as much time as you like, and use in the same way as you would use a gua sha stone (for example, in upward motions along the jawline). You do not need to rinse it off and can continue with your usual skincare routine after your cucumber facial is complete.

03 When you're finished, slice off the end that you've used so that the cucumber is clean and fresh for your next facial, and return it to the freezer.

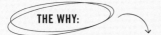

THE WHY:

- Cucumber is great for combating acne and breakouts, and can also help to reduce puffiness around the eyes and brighten dark circles. This frozen facial makes a wonderful aftersun treatment if you've accidentally rouged your skin!

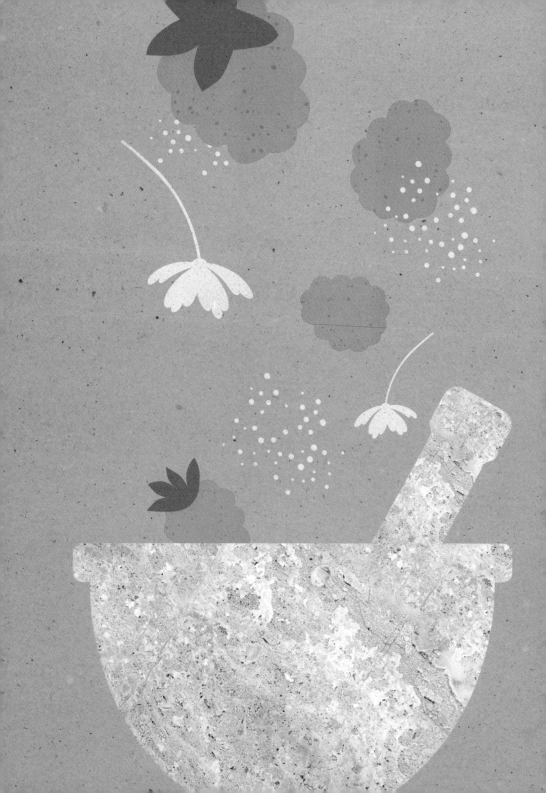

BEAUTY

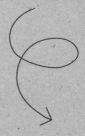

I've never loved that the beauty industry is called the beauty industry. If I critically think about it I'm not sure that 'the industry' has the same definition of beauty that I do. Things are certainly moving in the right direction, but when I was at my most impressionable as a teen, products were ONLY marketed by people who looked nothing like me. I feel passionately that my 'beauty' brand doesn't actually make people feel worse about themselves. Undoubtedly, the best part of my job is receiving images of skin transformations with incredible testimonials. Confidence can come from all sorts of things, but knowing that the products that I've designed have made so many feel that little bit more confident is the best feeling ever. Skincare and make-up have also been considered as separate categories until much more recent times. One of the main features of most make-up is that it's designed to stay on for long periods, so shouldn't we be making sure it's also nourishing our skin at the same time? I think so...

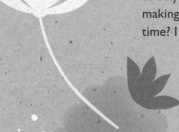

RASPBERRY LIP STAIN

MAKES 3 OR 4 USES

INGREDIENTS:

5–6 raspberries
1 teaspoon melted coconut oil

YOU WILL NEED:

pestle and mortar
fine-mesh strainer
small jar with a lid

TIP:

Want a deeper shade? Swap out the raspberries for blackberries!

Just like bags of salad, I find that raspberries turn a little mushy quite fast! This lip stain is a great way to make use of those berries so they don't end up getting binned. This simple lip stain creates a natural, flushed look. I shared this recipe on Instagram and TikTok and, at the time of writing, it was the most popular post we have ever made on both platforms. Who would've thought?! It also looks and tastes gorgeous - just resist licking it all off immediately!

01 Crush your raspberries using a pestle and mortar. Add the coconut oil and continue mashing it all together. Strain through a mesh strainer, then pour the strained mixture into your chosen container. Store in the fridge — this will keep for 3–5 days.

02 To use, simply dip your clean finger into the stain and apply to your lips.

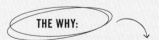

THE WHY:

- We've all learned the hard way that most berries stain pretty much everything – carpets, clothes, upholstery, the lot! So let's reclaim what's usually an irritating characteristic of this delicious fruit for something positive. Let's let it stain something we want staining!

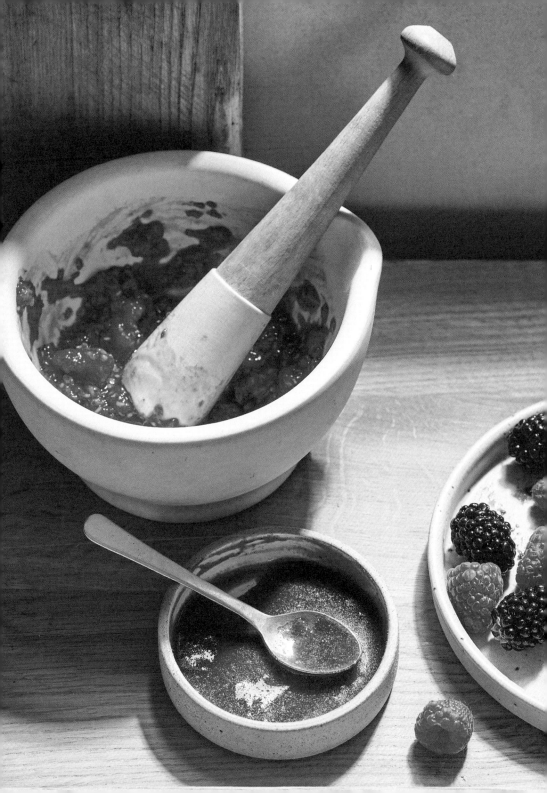

DEODORANT

**MAKES APPROX. 100 G
(3½ FL OZ)**

INGREDIENTS:

2 tablespoons melted coconut oil
2 tablespoons melted shea butter
2 tablespoons cornflour
(cornstarch)
3 tablespoons bicarbonate of soda
(baking soda) or arrowroot
2–3 drops of your fave essential
oil (see tip)

YOU WILL NEED:

glass jar with a lid
mini spatula or scoop

Say NO to BO (forgive me, I couldn't help myself!) with this quick and easy natural deodorant. In just a few simple steps you will be on your way to nourished, hydrated and fresh pits! Shea butter and coconut oil work to nourish the underarms, while bicarbonate of soda is pH-neutralising and antibacterial. Please note, this ingredient can be an irritant for some skin types, so I recommend doing a patch test first! Arrowroot can be used as an alternative for those who do not get on well with bicarbonate of soda.

01 Mix all the ingredients together in a bowl. Pour the mixture into a clean empty jar of your choice. Pop the lid on and leave it to sit for about 3–4 hours. This recipe will last for 6 months, stored sealed at room temperature, as it does not contain water, but you'll likely use it up before then if using regularly.

02 To use, portion yourself some deodorant with a mini spatula or scoop and apply it directly to the skin. This deodorant not only smells wonderful, but it's also 100 per cent natural and deeply moisturising.

TIP:

My two fave essential oil combos
to use here are tea tree and
orange, or lavender and patchouli.
If you want to make your own
Orange Peel Oil, see page 135.

THE WHY:

- Although they no longer contain the harmful chlorofluorocarbons (CFCs) that deplete the ozone layer, aerosol deodorants still contain gas propellants that contribute to air pollution and climate change.

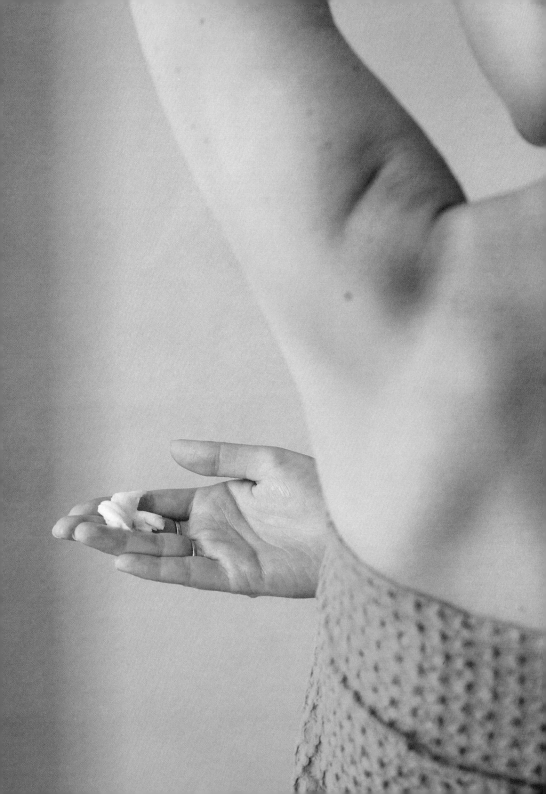

COCONUT OIL MAKE-UP REMOVER

INGREDIENTS:

coconut oil – that's it!

This is no longer a natural beauty enthusiast secret – in fact, I think it's fairly widespread knowledge these days – but all you need to remove make-up, including mascara, is coconut oil.

01 Simply warm a little coconut oil between your fingertips before applying to your face and eyelids. Massage in gently to lift off the make-up. Wipe away with a damp muslin, reusable make-up pad or face cloth.

ALOE +ROSE PRIMER

MAKES 15–20 USES

INGREDIENTS:

2 tablespoons aloe vera gel *(see page 139 for how to extract aloe gel from a leaf)*
2 tablespoons rose water *(see Rose Water Face Mist on page 68)*

YOU WILL NEED:

reusable bottle with a pump lid

This hydrating primer gives you a smooth and nourished base, making your make-up last longer and giving you a radiant look.

01 In a small bowl, combine the aloe vera gel and rose water. Carefully pour the mixture into your bottle. Ensure the lid is securely closed to prevent contamination and maintain freshness. Store in the fridge, where it keeps for 2–3 weeks. Doing so also helps my skin feel firm after application.

02 To use, cleanse your face and pat it dry. Take a small amount of primer and apply it all over your face using your fingertips or a make-up brush. Focus on areas that get oily or where make-up tends to fade quickly.

03 Allow the primer to set for a minute or two before applying foundation or any other make-up products.

THE WHY:

- Aloe vera is well known for its soothing and moisturising properties, while rose water helps to balance and hydrate the skin.

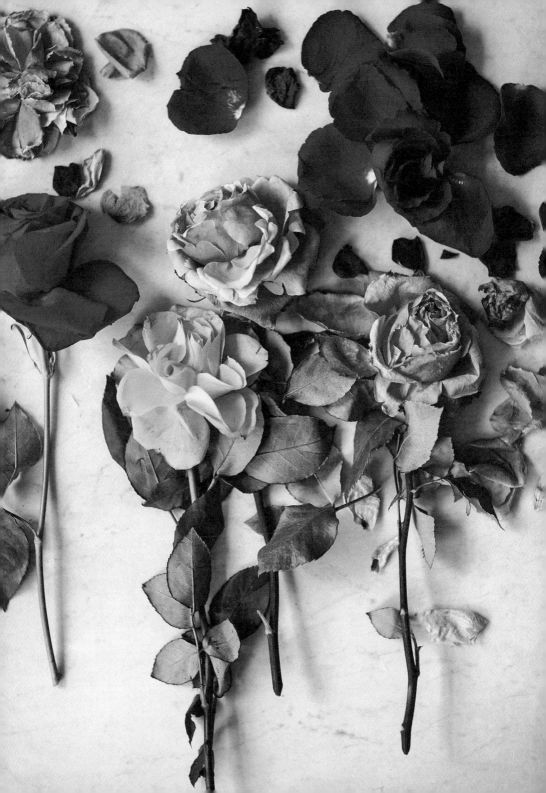

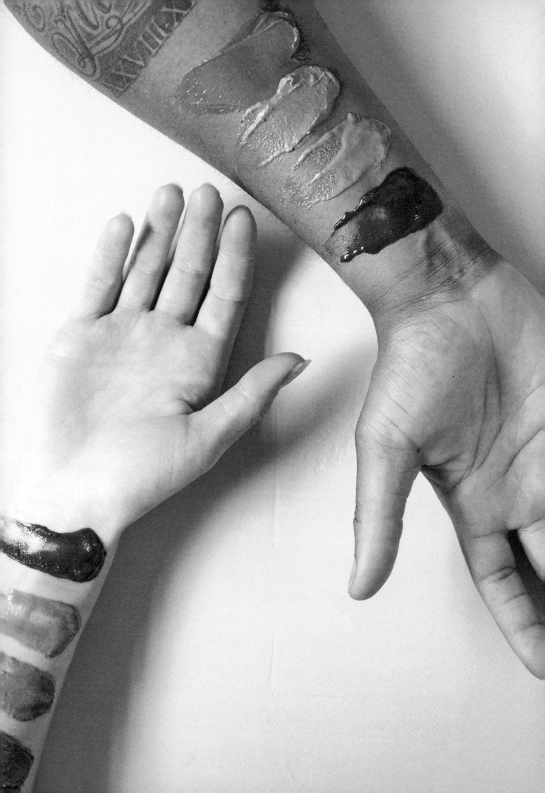

EYE SHADOW

MAKES ABOUT 15 G (½ OZ)

INGREDIENTS:

1 teaspoon ground turmeric
1 teaspoon cacao powder
1 teaspoon shea butter, melted

YOU WILL NEED:

small glass jar with a lid

TIP:

Whatever powders you use, make sure everything is very finely ground.

NOTE:

You could add some mica powder for a little shimmer. Be sure to purchase only mica powder that is for cosmetic use and safe to use near your eyes.

You can use any pigmented natural powder to create eye shadows in various shades, but your eyes are sensitive, so please carefully look into whether or not they're listed as safe for use on delicate skin. I've suggested some other options below, but here I'm going to be sharing a recipe for a sunshine-yellow shade – my favourite colour in the world. You might be thinking, 'Surely a powder like turmeric will stain my skin?' But rest assured, this should not happen after the powder is mixed with oils. Staining only occurs if it's applied neat. This eye shadow is easy to make, blends smoothly and moisturises your eyelids, too! I suggest doing a patch test and taking care if you do decide to give this a try! Also, we recommend applying over a base, such as primer, concealer or foundation.

01 Combine your powders in a small bowl, then stir in the melted shea butter. Transfer into your chosen jar, seal, and leave to set until solid.

02 It will keep for a year if stored in a sealed container and stored in a cool, dry place.

03 To use, swish a make-up brush gently over the surface before applying it to your eyelids.

RECOMMENDED POWDERS FOR OTHER SHADES:

- **Purple/blue** – freeze-dried blueberry powder
- **Pink** – freeze-dried raspberry powder, hibiscus powder or beetroot powder
- **Green** – spirulina or moringa powder
- **Orange/yellow** – ground turmeric
- **Brown** – cacoa powder
- **White** – kaolin clay
- **Dusty rose** – rose kaolin clay
- **Light green** – French green clay

BEETROOT CHEEK TINT

**MAKES APPROX. 10 G
(¼ OZ) – ABOUT 30 USES**

INGREDIENTS:

1 teaspoon of Beetroot Powder
 (see page 138)
1 teaspoon arrowroot powder

YOU WILL NEED:

glass jar with a lid

This cheek tint has only two - yes, two - ingredients. I've always been more of a fan of the bronzy look than pink, but as with most of the recipes in this book, you can swap out certain ingredients to create different results. For example, dragon fruit powder creates a pink blush, cacao powder gives a deeper brown, the beetroot that I use creates a reddish brown, and you can even get purple sweet potato powder that, as you can imagine, is a beautiful violet hue. Here, I've also shown you how to make your own beetroot powder on page 138, which you can then use in the tint.

01 First, make the beetroot powder on page 138.

02 Combine the two powders in a clean, thoroughly dry jar using a clean utensil like a chopstick. To adjust the shade of the blush, you can add more beetroot powder, or more arrowroot for a lighter shade.

02 It will keep for a year in a sealed container and stored in a cool, dry place.

03 To use, gently dip your make-up brush in the mixture and use the edge of the jar to tap off the excess back into the jar, then gently apply to the cheeks.

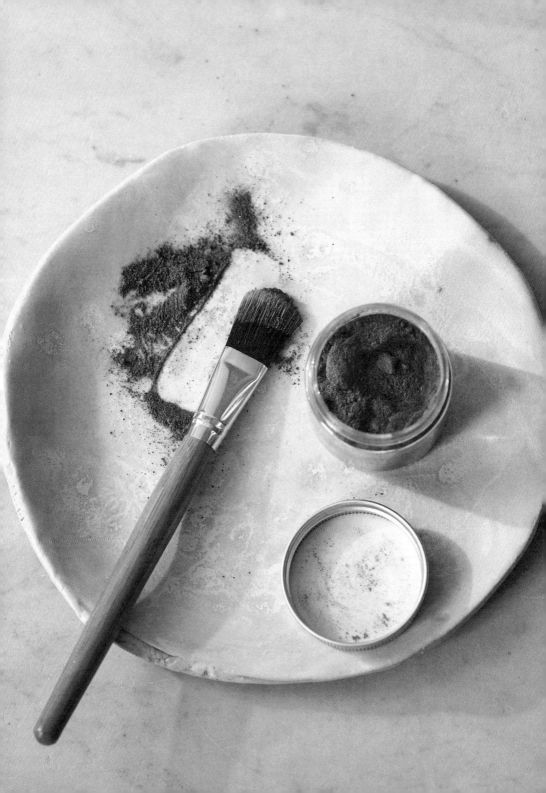

MASCARA
(doubles as an eyebrow tint)

**MAKES ABOUT 10 ML
(¹/₃ FL OZ)**

INGREDIENTS:

pinch of bentonite clay
generous pinch of activated
  charcoal *(for black mascara)* or
  cocoa powder *(for brown)* – if your
  activated charcoal is in capsule
  form, then 1 capsule should
  be plenty
5 drops of vitamin E oil
5 drops of castor oil
5 drops of vegetable glycerine
½ teaspoon of aloe vera gel *(see
  page 139 for how to extract aloe gel
  from a leaf)*

YOU WILL NEED:

wide, shallow jar with a lid
  (see tip)
mascara wand

TIP:

*Choose a very shallow container
that'll allow you to swipe the
long edge of your mascara wand
across the surface. If the lip of
the container is too high, or the
mouth is too narrow, then you'll
only be able to dip the tip of your
wand into it! You're better off with
a wide, shallow container than a
tall, narrow one!*

My biggest pet peeve with mascara is that so many of them crumble a little onto the cheeks after more than 3 or 4 hours of wear. Given this, it seems like they're not so good at staying on, but then when it comes to actually removing it I still lose a lash or two in my attempts to get it all off. What I like most about this DIY version is that it stays on your lashes whilst you want it there and comes off when you don't!

01 Mix the dry ingredients in a bowl or directly in the container you'll be using to store your mascara. I use a chopstick to mix. Add the wet ingredients and stir thoroughly. Allow to set for an hour or so before applying.

02 It will keep for 6 months if stored in a sealed container in a cool, dry place. Close the container as soon as you've used it in order to retain the moisture of the mascara for as long as possible.

03 To use, simply use a clean mascara wand to apply to your lashes.

THE WHY:

- Both vitamin E and castor oil are thought to promote lash growth, and vitamin E also works as a natural preservative, helping your mascara to last longer.

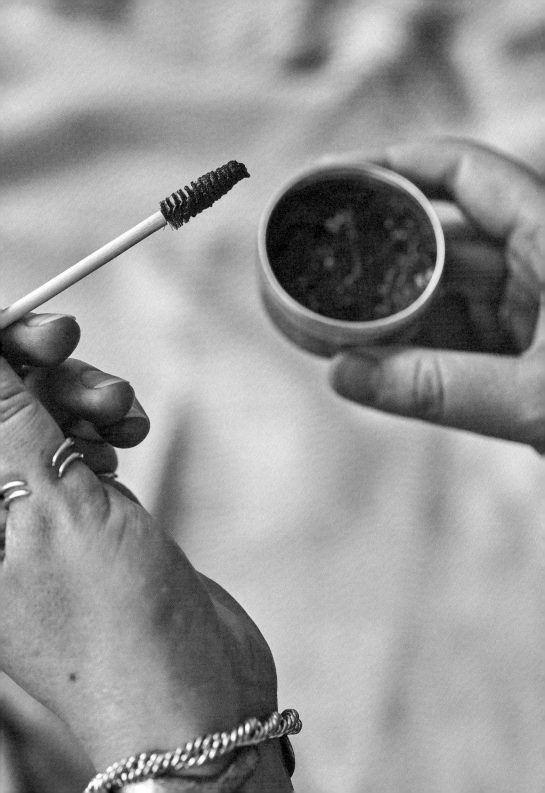

DRY SHAMPOO

**MAKES APPROX. 20–30 G
(¾–1 OZ)** / *about 10 uses,
depending on the length of
your hair*

INGREDIENTS:

1 tablespoon cornflour *(cornstarch)*
or finely blended oats
1 tablespoon your chosen powder:
· *blonde* – arrowroot
· *red* – cinnamon
· *brunette* – cocoa or cacao
powder
· *black* – ground charcoal
· *dyed pink, green, blue, etc.*
– crushed coloured chalk in a
matching colour

YOU WILL NEED:

glass jar, ideally with a shaker lid

The aim of a dry shampoo is to instantly absorb excess oil from your hair. This DIY version is an absolute essential if you're packing light, off to a festival or simply looking for some extra oomph for your hair between washes. As the base, you can use either cornflour (cornstarch), which is great for absorbing oil and grease, or very finely blended oats, which also absorb excess oil, but are also good for more irritated or itchy scalps. Further ingredients will need to be chosen based on your hair colour.

01 Simply combine your chosen base powder with your chosen colour powder. If you're somewhere in the middle, like me, you can mix and match the colour powders to get the right shade, as if they were paint. I'm either a very dark blonde or a light brunette, so I use a bit of arrowroot and a bit of cocoa powder. Once you're happy with the shade, transfer to your jar.

02 It will keep for a year if stored in a sealed container in a cool, dry place.

03 If you use a jar with a shaker lid, you can just apply directly to your hair as needed! Otherwise, dip a make-up brush or clean paintbrush into the powder and gently brush it onto your roots until no more powder is visible.

THE WHY:

• This natural powder does not contain the alcohol and drying agents that many shop-bought dry shampoos contain. Scalps can be sensitive, so applying lots of different chemicals can exacerbate this. Using this dry shampoo means you can delay washing your hair by a day or two; over time, this means you'll need to wash your hair less often, helping to balance oil levels naturally.

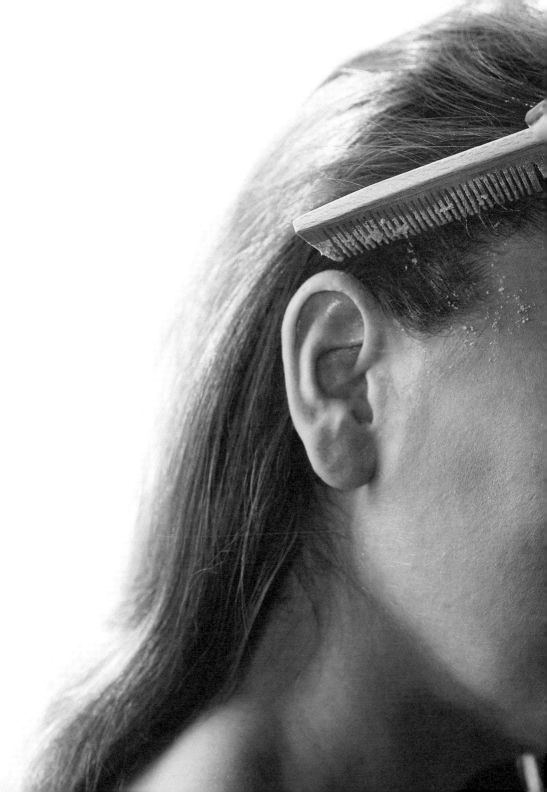

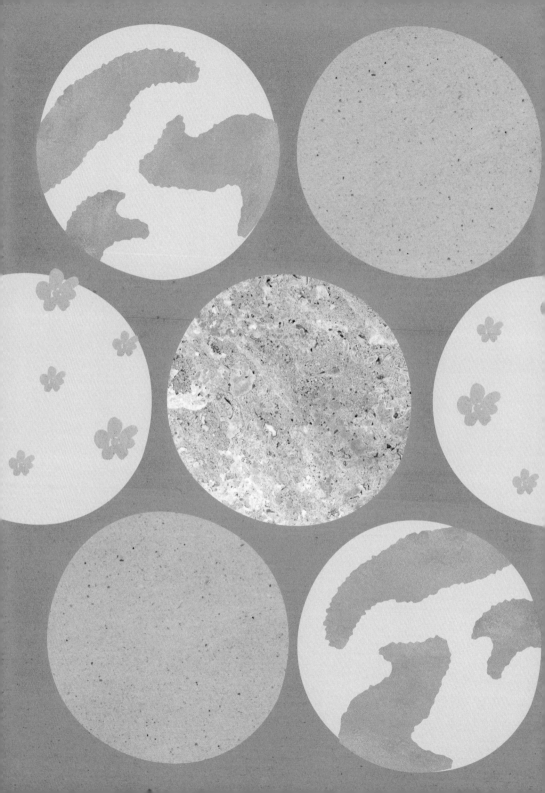

BATH BITS

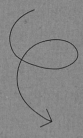

I only really take baths in the winter, so when I do, I like to really go for it. This is probably because if I say 'I think I need a bath' it's usually more about mentally needing a bath than physically needing one. These recipes are all about creating an atmosphere of relaxation. So, enjoy the process of making them, then sink into warm, beautifully scented water and unwind!

BATH SALTS

MAKES ABOUT 400 G (14 OZ)
enough for about 20 baths

INGREDIENTS:

4 or 5 flowerheads past their best
350–400 g *(12–14 oz)* sea salt,
Epsom salt and/or Himalayan
pink salts *(this is the trio of
dreams, but you don't have to use
all three)*
8–9 drops of your fave essential
oils *(our suggestions include
orange, rose, geranium and
lavender)*

YOU WILL NEED:

large jar with a lid – a big pickle or
jam jar works nicely, or a Kilner
jar brings a nice aesthetic

TIP:
*These salts make a great gift.
Reuse a pretty jar and paint it in
the recipient's favourite colours,
or match it to the colour scheme
of their bathroom!*

Bath salts have been around forever, but they often don't get the appreciation they deserve. Submerging your body in a bath filled with warm water and salt is proven to be one of the best ways to restore yourself after a long day. This health-promoting ritual soothes the muscles, hydrates the skin, detoxifies the body and can relieve internal swelling.

The story behind the bath salts in our range truly sums up what UpCircle as a brand is all about. We use a railway arch as a warehouse, and all our neighbours are florists. I noticed over time that on the same day each week, the bins outside each arch would be brimming with BEAUTIFUL flowers. These were flowers that had not been sold the week prior, and therefore did not have a long-enough shelf life to be sold on. So, I asked all my neighbours if they'd be willing to let us have those unloved stems instead. This is where the idea for our bath salts was born. We released the final product one year later! This is pretty much the exact recipe for them...

01 Separate your petals from their buds/stems. Spread them out on a baking tray and dehydrate them in your oven on a very low heat (about 100°C/210°F/gas ¼) for about 20 minutes. You'll know they're done when they're completely crispy. The idea is to remove all moisture from the leaves. They should turn a darker shade of their original colour (not brown or black). Crumble the crispy petals into little flakes.

02 In a bowl, combine your salts before mixing in the essential oils and petals. Transfer to your chosen jar.

03 To use, pour the equivalent of about 2 heaped tablespoons of salts into your bath and enjoy!

THE WHY:

- The combination of the three different salts we have suggested here creates the most revitalising bathing experience. The macro and trace minerals found in the salts are necessary for our health and can actually be drawn into the bloodstream during a warm bath, which can help to balance out the entire body. Soaking in a warm salt solution for 15–20 minutes provides great benefits in terms of improving the skin barrier function, hydrating the skin, and decreasing inflammation.

BATH BOMBS
three ways

MAKES 3 BATH BOMBS

INGREDIENTS:

90 g *(3 oz)* 6 tablespoons
  bicarbonate of soda *(baking soda)*
45 g *(2 oz)* 3 tablespoons citric acid
30 g *(1 oz)* 3 tablespoons cornflour
  (cornstarch)
45 g *(2 oz)* 3 tablespoons
  Epsom salt
2 tablespoons olive oil or coconut oil
mica powder colouring in your
  chosen colour *(or, if that's too
  much of a faff, then food colouring
  also does the job nicely – just use a
  few drops per bomb)*, optional

TO MAKE CITRUS BATH BOMBS:
3 drops of orange essential oil or
  Orange Peel Oil *(page 135)*
peel of 1 satsuma/tangerine

TO MAKE LAVENDER BATH BOMBS:
3 drops of lavender essential oil
5–10 lavender buds that have fallen
  from the sprigs

TO MAKE ROSE BATH BOMBS:
3 drops of rose essential oil
5–10 'past their best' rose petals
  dried in the oven

YOU WILL NEED:

silicone bath bomb moulds *(see tip)*

Who doesn't love a bath bomb?! There are the scents, the colours and even the sound as they fizz to nothing, and the beauty of the petals they leave floating on the water – they satisfy every sense, and truly elevate your bathing experience. I LOVE this little trio of bath bombs; they look gorgeous and make a super-easy gift too. Either choose your favourite 'flavour' or make all three.

01 In a bowl, mix together the baking soda, citric acid, cornflour and Epsom salt.

02 In a smaller bowl, combine the olive or coconut oil with your essential oil, as well as the food colouring, if using.

03 Slowly incorporate the wet ingredients with the dry. If you're using mica powder to colour your mixture, add that now. If your mixture is still very dry (you're aiming for it to be a bit clumpy), add a few drops of water – the mixture will fizz, so you'll need to whisk it in very quickly.

04 If you're using citrus peel, lay some pieces of peel in your moulds, trying to lie them quite flat so they end up on the surface of the bomb. The flower petals can be mixed into the bowl with the rest of the ingredients rather than lining the mould.

05 If you're adding colour, and making one of each variety, split your mixture into 3 at this stage and add the colour to each mix independently.

06 Fill your moulds with the bath bomb mixture and try to compact it as much as you can. Use the back of a spoon to smooth out the surface if you're using an ice-cube tray as your mould.

07 Leave to set for 3–6 hours.

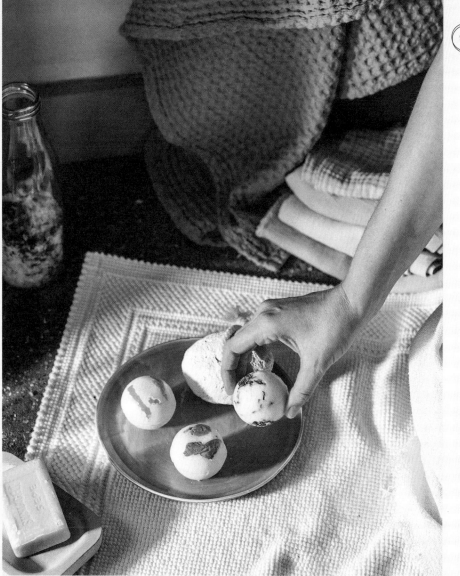

Large silicone ice-cube trays, cupcake trays, yogurt pots or cookie cutters work for this; just be sure to really pack your mixture down into the space to help the bombs keep their shape.

08 Carefully remove the bath bombs from the moulds, and they are ready to use! Make sure they stay dry until you're ready to use them – they will last up to 6 months if stored properly.

09 To use, drop into a bath of warm water!

SAGE BATH OIL

MAKES 75 ML (3 FL OZ)
enough for about 15 baths

INGREDIENTS:

5–20 wilted or 'past their best' sage leaves
75 ml *(3 fl oz)* olive or almond oil

YOU WILL NEED:

glass jar
saucepan
fine-mesh strainer or a piece of muslin *(cheesecloth)*
glass bottle or jar with a lid

> **TIP:**
> *Before adding any oils to your bath, make sure you close the bathroom door so that you can keep as much of the scent in the room as possible.*

The aroma of essential or scented oils is so much stronger in warm water. It's almost like sniffing a bunch of flowers. The scent of herbs gives me instant spa vibes, so here I'll be making my own sage oil. I have sage growing in my garden, so I make my oil from any leaves that have imperfections or that I wouldn't choose to cook with.
If sage isn't your vibe, you can use another homemade oil, like the Apricot Kernel Oil on page 136, the Orange Peel Oil on page 135, the Lemon Peel Oil on page 134, or the Mint-infused Oil on page 132. Alternatively, you can just dilute your favourite essential oil in a carrier oil – see the note on page 102.

01 Begin by ensuring the sage leaves are clean and free of any dirt or debris. Rinse them gently under cold water and pat them dry, then leave them to wilt for a few hours to reduce the water content, as excess moisture can cause the oil to spoil more quickly.

02 Place the wilted sage leaves in your glass jar, then pour over the oil; it should be enough to fully cover them. Gently stir the mixture to remove any air bubbles.

03 Fill the saucepan with about 7.5 cm (3 in) water and place over a very low heat. Place your glass jar into the water, ensuring that the surrounding water does not come over the top and spill into the oil. Leave for 1–2 hours, but check it regularly to ensure the oil doesn't get too hot – you don't want it to reach a simmer.

04 After the infusion period is over, leave the oil to cool, then strain it into a clean, dry bowl. This will remove the wilted sage leaves and any sediment, leaving you with a clear, aromatic, sage-infused oil.

05 Transfer the homemade sage oil into a clean, airtight glass bottle or jar. Store in a cool, dark place, such as a kitchen or bathroom cupboard. Properly stored, the sage oil can last for several months. However, always check for any signs of spoilage before use.

06 To use, run a bath and add 5 drops of your homemade bath oil. Put on your favourite music, lie back and enjoy!

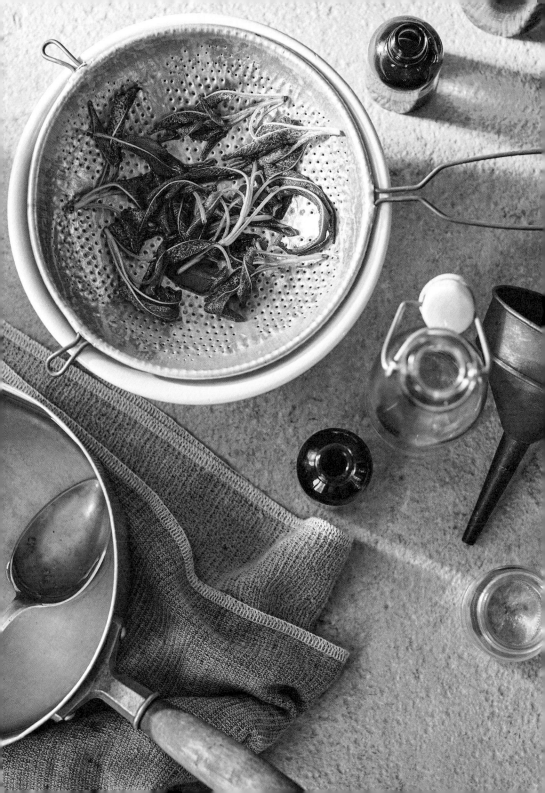

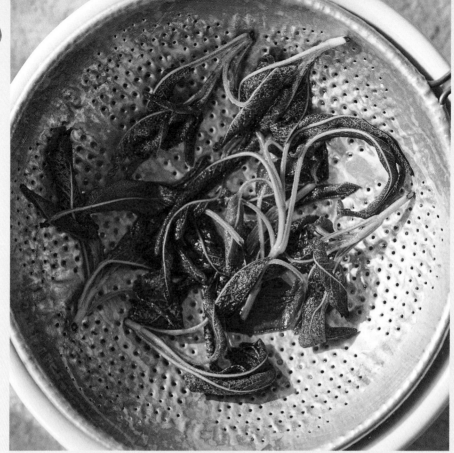

BATHING IN ESSENTIAL OILS

The basic principle when adding essential oils to a bath is to select essential oils for their properties and fragrance, then add them to your chosen base carrier oil. We suggest using a light base oil as your carrier oil, such as almond oil, jojoba oil, grapeseed oil, or even simple olive oil. Usually, you will need about 10 drops of essential oil, which you can add to 1 tablespoon of your chosen carrier oil and then use in your bath, but with some of the stronger-smelling oils (such as eucalyptus, peppermint, bay, basil, lime, lemon, thyme and rosemary) you will only need 5 drops.

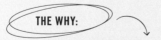

THE WHY:

- Because sage is more spa-like than any other oil, and everyone deserves to feel like they've been transported to a spa when they have a bath at home!

SIMPLE PEBBLE FOOT BATH

MAKES ABOUT 230 ML (7½ FL OZ)

Feet need some love too! This is a great recipe for anyone wanting to pamper them the way they should be pampered!

INGREDIENTS:

5 drops of Sage Oil *(see page 100)* or your favourite essential oil

YOU WILL NEED:

enough smooth pebbles to cover the base of your chosen bowl *(see tip)*
bowl or tub big enough to soak your feet, such as a washing-up bowl

01 To start, make your own homemade sage oil by following the instructions on page 100.

02 Ensure that the pebbles are clean. Then, place the pebbles in your chosen tub or bowl and fill it with warm water. Add your chosen essential oil and give the water a quick swish around to help it disperse.

03 Start by letting your feet soak in the water for a few minutes, then begin to move your feet around the pebbles, going back and forth.

04 Relax your feet in the water for as long as you like; I usually do this for about 20–30 minutes! This is a mini self-care ritual I love to do before a holiday.

TIP:

If you don't have any pebbles, marbles are a good substitute.

THE WHY:

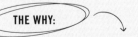

• This massage feels wonderful and you'll quickly feel it simulating all your reflexology zones.

HOME

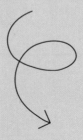

Homewares tend to be very expensive, but they're also usually incredibly simple to make at home from items that you'll already have – like flower petals! Throwing away flowers that are starting to look a bit sad makes me feel sad, so I always find a way to use them once they start to wilt and fade. Lots of the recipes in this section also make gorgeous little gifts – they have real 'wow' factor, but most take about five minutes to make!

DRAWER FRESHENER

MAKES 1

INGREDIENTS:

bunch of flowers that are 'past their best'
4 tablespoons rice or coffee beans
5-10 drops of your favourite essential oil *(see tip)*

YOU WILL NEED:

small cotton drawstring bag/pouch

TIPS:

1. If you're using rice, any essential oils will work well. The rice simply acts as a holding agent for the scent that you add. If you use coffee beans, they have a strong scent, so choose an oil that will pair well with coffee, such as cinnamon, peppermint, orange, ginger, cardamom or lavender.

2. Used tea bags are also good for neutralising odours anywhere in your home. Simply place (dry) used tea bags into a mesh bag/ pouch and pop the bag at the back of your fridge, in your car, or wherever! I use 4–5 tea bags in the bag at a time and replace them every 5 days.

Smell the roses – and the coffee – and whatever you want, really! This super-easy drawer freshener is a great way to keep your clothes smelling fresher for longer. And it's not just about your draw-dwelling delicates, this can be adapted to keep hanging items smelling great, too – just use the strings of the pouch to tie this onto the hanging rail in your wardrobe.

01 De-petal your flowers, then spread them out on a baking tray and dehydrate them in your oven set to a very low heat (about 100°C/210°F/gas ¼) for about 20 minutes. You'll know they're done when they're completely crispy. The idea is to remove all moisture from the petals.

02 Tip the rice or coffee beans into a bowl and add your chosen essential oil. Allow the oil to fully absorb into the rice or coffee before tipping into your drawstring bag – the mixture should not look or feel at all wet.

03 Add the dried-out petals, give the bag a little shake, then pull the strings tightly to close the pouch and pop it in your drawer or hang from the rail in your wardrobe. When the scent fades, simply add more drops of essential oil to the rice or coffee!

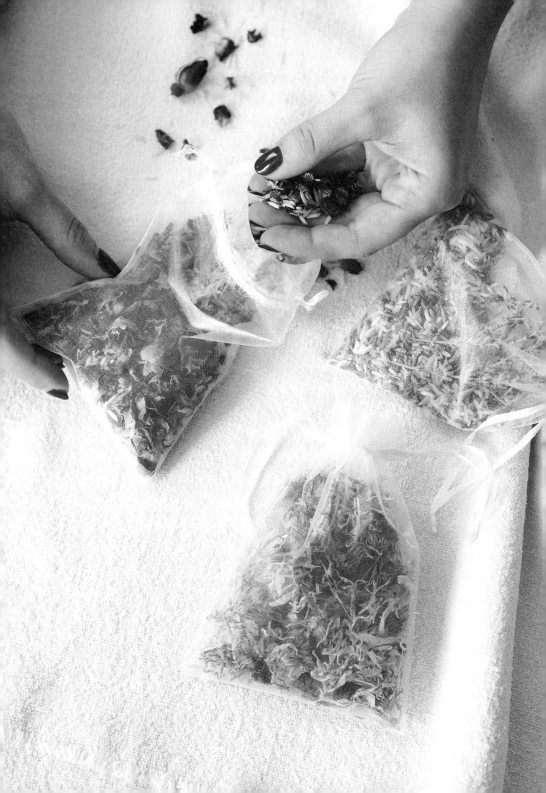

CITRUS SURFACE-CLEANING SPRAY

**MAKES ABOUT
200–300 ML (7–10 FL OZ)**

INGREDIENTS:

peels of about 5 citrus fruits –
   lemons, limes, grapefruits,
   oranges or a combination!
200–300 ml *(7-10 fl oz)* white wine
   vinegar
2–3 browning rosemary sprigs
   (optional)

YOU WILL NEED:

glass jar with a sealable lid - Kilner
   jars work well as they have a
   rubber seal around the lid
fine-mesh strainer
spray bottle *(reuse an empty one)*

When life gives you lemons... make a natural all-purpose cleaner! If you've made fresh grapefruit juice, or been enjoying lots of oranges or satsumas, don't throw away the peels. This spray works well on kitchen and bathroom surfaces because the acidic nature of vinegar helps to break down dirt, grease and grime whilst the citrus fruits neutralise odours and have antibacterial properties.

01 Place all your citrus peels into the jar, then pour over the vinegar. Make sure all the peels are submerged to avoid mould. Seal the jar and leave to sit for 2–3 weeks in a sunny spot.

02 Strain the liquid and transfer to your spray bottle. If you find the vinegar scent off-putting then adding a couple of sprigs of rosemary works really well. Alternatively, if your spray bottle isn't completely full you can top it up with water to dilute the scent. This will keep at room temperature for 3 months.

03 To use, simply spray on your surfaces and wipe.

THE WHY:

• Vinegar is a great disinfectant, and most citrus fruits have both antibacterial and anti-microbial properties.

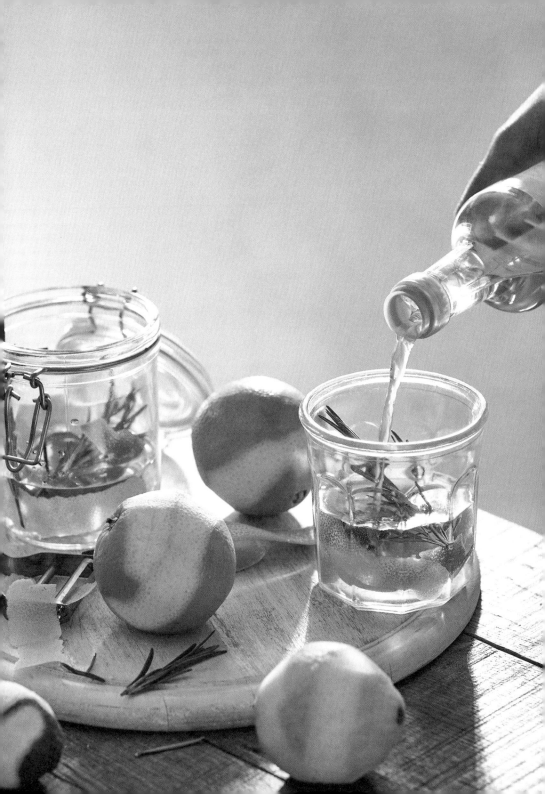

ALL-PURPOSE CLEANER

THE MANY, MANY USES FOR RICE WATER

Now, before we even get into this, I'd like to start by saying that I am aware you're not supposed to have lots of water leftover when making rice. But, let's be honest, it can be tricky to nail it 100 per cent of the time. I've always been a bit useless at getting ratios and quantities spot on - plus, depending on the sort of rice, its starch content, and several other factors, cooking rice is far from an exact science. So, if you end up with leftover rice water after cooking, or are someone who likes to rinse rice during the cooking process, here are three ways that you can use that water around your home rather than just pouring it away.

- **Use it to clean your dishes** – Rice water is great at breaking down grease and oil.
- **Use it to polish glass or mirrors** – Rice water is starchy and slightly acidic, which is why it works so well on smears and foggy-looking glass.
- **Use it to water your plants** – The starches in rice water provide plants with carbohydrates that can be stored in the plant's cell membrane until they can be used for energy. It also promotes healthy bacteria population within the soil and acts as an organic method of pest control. It can be applied through top watering, bottom watering or misting.

And it's not just useful around the home - rice water can also be a valuable tool in your beauty kit.

- **Use it like a cleanser and then rinse off** – Rice water can help keep spots at bay. It also contains many antioxidants, which can help skin to retain its elasticity.
- **Use it as a hair rinse** – A rice water rinse can have particular benefits for those with curls – it really makes them pop. Rice water also contains B vitamins and vitamin E, which help to give hair shine and improve its strength, preventing breakages and split ends.

CONDITIONER BAR
FABRIC SPRAY

INGREDIENTS:

conditioner bar scraps

YOU WILL NEED:

spray bottle

You've bought or been gifted this book, so the chances are you've come across or used a solid conditioner before. This recipe is much like the Soap-scrap Make-up Brush Cleaner on page 120, but uses the scraps from a conditioner bar as opposed to a soap or shampoo bar. It has a similar effect on fabric as a conditioner has on your hair; it softens it and leaves a delicate fresh scent.

01 All you need to do is add your conditioner scraps to a bowl of warm water. As a guide, the approximate ratio should be nine parts water to one part conditioner. Leave it until the scraps dissolve and melt into the water. Depending on the brand of conditioner bar, you may need to heat the mixture a little, which you can do in the microwave for 20 seconds or in a bain-marie.

02 Once it's ready, decant into a spray bottle and go wild — I spray this on my sofa, blankets, bedsheets, guest towels — you name it!

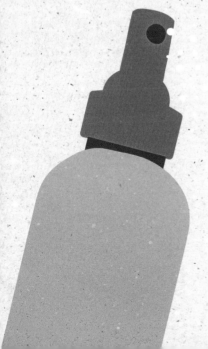

CHAMOMILE PILLOW MIST

MAKES 250 ML (8 FL OZ)

INGREDIENTS:

3-4 used chamomile tea bags
250 ml *(8 fl oz)* water – ideally
    filtered or distilled
1 tablespoon witch hazel
5–6 drops of lavender essential oil,
    or any other calming essential oil

YOU WILL NEED:

saucepan
spray bottle

TIP:

*Before using the pillow mist, it's
a good idea to test it on a small
area of your pillow to check for
any discolouration or staining
(although this is unlikely with
chamomile and lavender).*

I've asked as many friends and family as I possibly can how long they leave their tea to steep before drinking. The average time was a minute and a half, with lots of people saying they leave a tea bag in the water for less than 60 seconds. This means there's still a lot of goodness left in the herbs or flowers inside your tea bag. So, let's make use of it! Indulge in a calming and sustainable bedtime routine with this chamomile pillow mist made from used chamomile tea bags. Chamomile is well known for its soothing and relaxing properties, making it the perfect natural ingredient to help you unwind and prepare for a restful night's sleep.

01 Ensure your tea bags are thoroughly dried. You can let them air-dry for a few hours or pop them in the oven on a very low heat (about 100°C/210°F/gas ¼) for 20–30 minutes to speed up the process.

02 Pour the water into a small saucepan and bring to a gentle boil over a medium heat. Once it reaches the boil, turn off the heat and add the dried chamomile tea bags. Let the tea bags steep for about 10–15 minutes, allowing the chamomile to infuse into the water. If you prefer a stronger scent, you can leave the tea bags in for a bit longer.

03 After the steeping time, remove the tea bags and allow the infusion to cool to room temperature.

04 Once the chamomile infusion has cooled, add the witch hazel. Witch hazel helps disperse the essential oil you'll be adding next and also gives the mist a longer shelf life.

05 Add the essential oil, then carefully pour the chamomile pillow mist into the spray bottle. Shake the bottle gently to ensure the essential oil is well distributed. Aim to use within 4–6 weeks for the scent to be at its best.

06 To use, spray a light mist over your pillow and bedding just before bedtime. Take a deep breath and enjoy the calming aroma of chamomile and lavender as you prepare for a peaceful night's sleep.

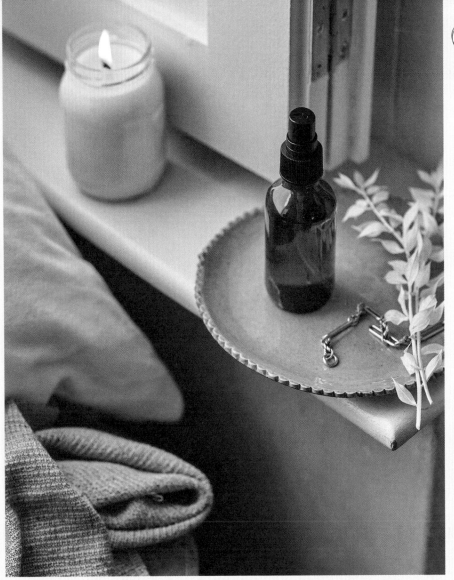

THE WHY:

- Chamomile is renowned for its calming effects, helping to reduce stress and anxiety, and promoting relaxation before bedtime. Its soothing aroma can help improve sleep quality and contribute to a more restful slumber, and this is complemented perfectly by the relaxing scent of lavender. By making your own pillow mist, you can ensure it's free from harmful chemicals and synthetic fragrances often found in commercial products. At UpCircle we upcycle chamomile stems into our Face Toner!

UPCYCLED CANDLE

MAKES 1 CANDLE

INGREDIENTS:

180 ml *(6 fl oz)* soy wax

2 teaspoons powdered upcycled ingredient of your choice *(make sure this complements the oils you've chosen - for example, cinnamon oil and ginger oil work brilliantly with any spice combo)*

15 drops of the essential oils of your choice

approx. 10 dried flower petals *(optional)* - see page 106 for how to dry out your petals

YOU WILL NEED:

an empty jar, the size of an average jar of jam

string suitable for acting as a wick - or you can purchase prepared wicks online very cheaply

heatproof bowl and saucepan to create a bain-marie/ double-boiler

clothes pegs

A very popular product in the UpCircle range is our Chai Latte candle, which is made with soy wax and infused with upcycled chai spices. The chai spices include fennel, cardamom, all spice, star anise, nutmeg, cloves and ginger. The chai company we're partnered with sources these organic spices from across the globe. They pour boiling water through them all to create chai syrups that they sell to the hospitality industry, but the delicious spices are leftover, so that's where we step in to save them! We dry them out, before grinding them into the most incredible aromatic powder.

If you make your own chai at home, then you can follow exactly same process on a smaller scale. But it doesn't have to be chai - similar spices are added to mulled wine! So keep the cloves and cinnamon sticks and you can dry them out for a spiced yet rich and fruity (from the wine and satsumas) scented powder. And it's not just spices - dried flower petals are also an excellent option and pair beautifully with any flower oil, such as rose, patchouli or ylang-ylang.

The process here is creative and experimental - you can play around with colours and scent combos, even dispersing textures through the wax or using moulds of different shapes. These make the loveliest gifts, particularly around Christmas, and you can make lots at once. Easy!

01 Start by preparing the jars. Place the wick into the jar, making sure the base of the wick is in the centre of the base of the jar. (You don't need glue, most come with a small cylinder of metal which helps to stabilise them.) The wick needs to have an extra 10 cm (4 in) sticking out from the top of the candle jar.

02 Fill the saucepan with about 5 cm (2 in) water and bring to a simmer over a medium heat. Place the heatproof bowl on top of the saucepan, ensuring it fits securely without touching the water. Add the wax to the bowl, stir gently and allow to melt over the course of about 5 minutes.

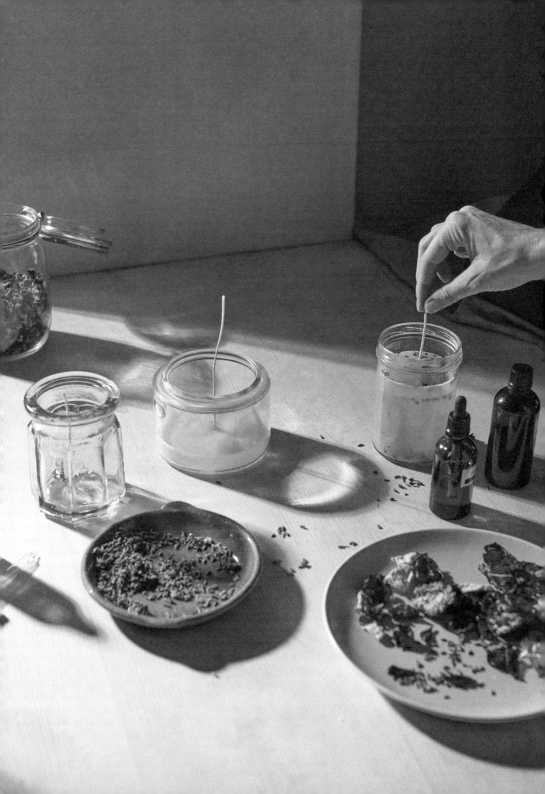

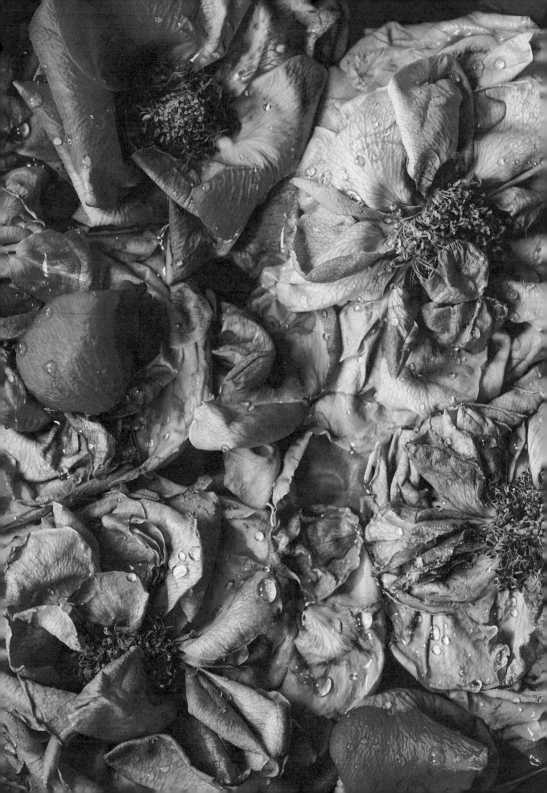

TIP:

If you have 4 or 5 nearly finished candles with a bit of wax left, don't throw them away – simply combine them! Place them all into a saucepan and pour water into the pan around them, making sure the water level is below the height of the candle jars (like a bain-marie). Place over a medium heat until the wax melts. Remove the old wicks, add new ones and pour the melted waxes into a new container (or your favourite of the old containers). Voilà - a new candle made from old candles!

03 Remove from the heat, then add about three-quarters of your upcycled powder, along with your chosen essential oil. If you're using petals, you can add these too – I'd recommend tearing them into smaller pieces and dispersing them sparingly through the wax, or else the petals will pool in the melted wax and interrupt the smoothness of the burn.

04 Carefully pour all of your mixture into the prepared jar. To make sure that the wick doesn't fall into the melted wax and become lost forever, clip it with a clothes peg and place the peg across the top of the jar to hold the wick upright as the wax sets.

05 Leave to set overnight.

06 Once set, or nearly set, sprinkle more of the repurposed ingredients on top. Finally, trim the wicks down to the desired length, and the candles are ready for their new homes!

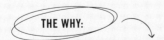

THE WHY:

- Making your own candles is an absolute bargain compared to the eye-watering prices of most candles on the market.

TWIG REED DIFFUSER

MAKES ONE DIFFUSER

INGREDIENTS:

8 tablespoons almond oil
1 tablespoon vodka
30 drops of essential oils *(combine these based on your preferences – some of my favourites are bergamot, jasmine, ylang-ylang, lavender and geranium)*

YOU WILL NEED:

small bundle of twigs *(see above)*
glass bottle with a narrow neck *(this will slow the evaporation of the liquid)*
ribbon or twine to decorate the bottle *(optional)* – natural twine in particular looks gorgeous with natural twigs/pine needles

Reed diffusers, in my opinion, tend to be either inexpensive but sickly sweet and artificial-smelling, or natural with well-blended scents, but incredibly pricey. There are a couple of recipes in this book that use petals from 'past their best' flower displays. Here, you can make use of the stems as the reeds for our diffuser oil. Alternatively, head out into your garden or local park to forage for some thin twigs! Some work better than others, so here's what to look for:

- *the stalks from perennials, such as echinacea or poppy stems*
- *long, thin, dead twigs – you shouldn't be breaking or pulling anything off anything!*
- *very long pine needles, bamboo sprigs or any light porous wood*

01 After gathering your twigs, leave them to dry out thoroughly for 2–3 days, or pop them into the oven set to a very low heat (about 100°C/210°F/gas ¼) for 30 minutes. Once dry, peel off the outer bark where possible.

02 Put the oil, vodka and essential oil(s) into your bottle and stir to combine. Place your twigs into the bottle, ensuring that they all reach the liquid. I swill the bottle around a little at this stage to kick things off a bit!

03 Place your diffuser in the room of your choice and enjoy! Once you can no longer smell the scent (usually after 2–3 weeks), flip the twigs the other way up. Overall, your diffuser should last you a month or so before you need to replace the oil and twigs.

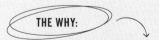 **THE WHY:**

- Twigs and stems naturally draw liquids upwards, so they're perfect for diffusing your oil out of the bottle and into your chosen room.

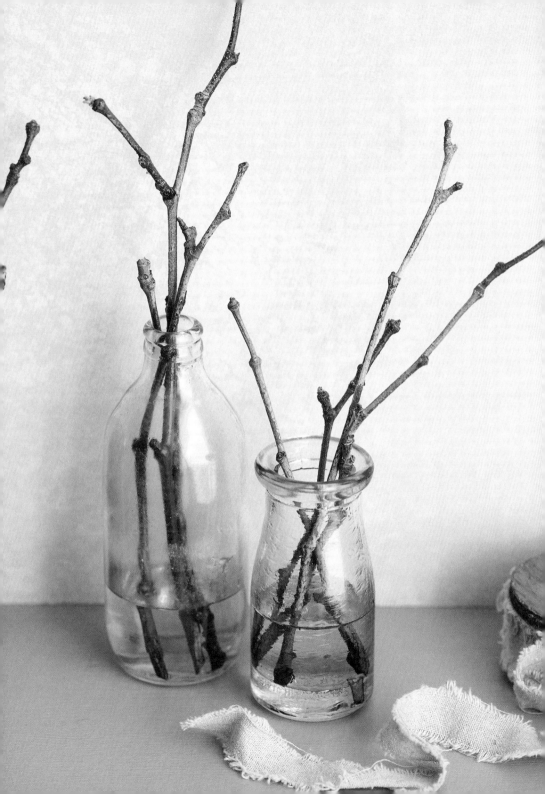

SOAP-SCRAP MAKE-UP BRUSH CLEANER

INGREDIENTS:

soap bar or shampoo bar scraps

YOU WILL NEED:

clean glass microwave-safe jar with a lid

Soap bars have made a comeback, and I am here for it. No longer considered boring and old-fashioned, soaps have re-established their well-deserved reputation as a top-tier ethical cleansing option. They're travel-friendly, long-lasting, versatile, visually appealing and SHOULD be packaged with no plastic in sight. The ONLY shortfall with a soap bar is that when you're down to the last scraps they end up flying all over the place, before finally breaking up into smaller and smaller pieces. When they get to this stage, retire them from the shower stall and let them start their next phase as make-up brush cleaners! You can also use shampoo bars for this.

01 Pop your soap scraps into your chosen jar and microwave on high in 20-second bursts, stirring between each one (I use a chopstick), until the soap is fully melted. (If your jar is not microwave-safe, put your scraps into a microwaveable bowl for this part, then pour into your jar after melting.)

02 Cover the jar with a tea towel or loosely place the lid on top to prevent dust getting in, then leave to set for 3–4 hours.

03 Once hard, you can simply twizzle your dirty brushes into the set soap to clean them, then rinse! After using, just pop the lid on and keep for your next clean!

THE WHY:

- Cleaning your make-up brushes regularly is important for both hygiene and performance reasons. The advice is that you should clean your make-up brushes once a week, but I would be lying if I said I did it once a month… In my defence, I only wear make-up once or twice a week! However often you get round to cleaning your brushes, this is an easy way to do it. Most soap bars are made without artificial fragrances, are antimicrobial, sulphate-free and antibacterial, so they're brilliant at getting rid of stubborn make-up build-up without damaging your brushes.

BUG REPELLENT

**MAKES APPROX.
150 ML (5 FL OZ)**

INGREDIENTS:

5 tablespoons water
5 tablespoons witch hazel
20 drops of eucalyptus oil
20 drops of citronella oil

YOU WILL NEED:

spray bottle

Don't let mosquitos or moths stop you living your best adventure-filled outdoor life. I can't lie to you and say that I'm a huge bug fan, but I also don't want to spray horrific toxic fumes into the air to completely obliterate them in a violent fashion. I'd like to repel them, not annihilate them. If you feel the same way, then try this out!

01 Simply mix all of the ingredients together and decant into a spray bottle.

02 To use, apply sparingly to exposed skin. Do not use on cuts, wounds or irritated skin and do not apply to areas around the eyes or mouth. My preference is to spray onto my clothing and into the air around me, rather than directly onto my skin.

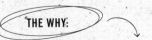 **THE WHY:**

- Something that I find very interesting is that citronella oil works by masking scents that are attractive to insects. It's for this reason that it repels rather than kills insects.

FABRIC DYE

**MAKES ENOUGH FOR
ONE SET OF BEDSHEETS
OR 5 T-SHIRTS**

INGREDIENTS:

3 small beetroots, peeled and diced
   into small pieces
big pinch of salt

FOR OTHER COLOURS:

YELLOW:
yellow onion skins

ORANGE:
carrot peel or butternut
   squash peel

INDIGO:
outer leaves of purple cabbage

YOU WILL NEED:

saucepan
fine-mesh strainer
large bowl or basin for dyeing
material

This recipe is less about upcycling the ingredients themselves, and more about reinventing clothing and linens. For example, you could transform a set of slightly stained or yellowed napkins by giving them a fresh fuchsia colour that looks good as new!

01 Tip the beetroot or other chosen colour ingredient into the saucepan and fill with boiling water. The more water you use, the less intense your shade of purple will be, so if you're only dyeing one t-shirt and want it to be a deeper shade, don't use too much water. Add the salt and bring to the boil over a medium heat. Continue to boil for 30–40 minutes – the water should become a deep red colour.

02 Strain the water into your bowl or basin through a fine-mesh strainer and allow to cool, then add your material and leave to soak for at least 3 hours.

03 After 3 hours, remove the material from the dye bath and gently squeeze to remove excess liquid. Allow to drip-dry overnight. Once it's thoroughly dried (I usually leave it a couple of days just so it's totally set in!) you can give it a quick wash in cool water by hand or in your machine, to be sure that no colour transfer occurs.

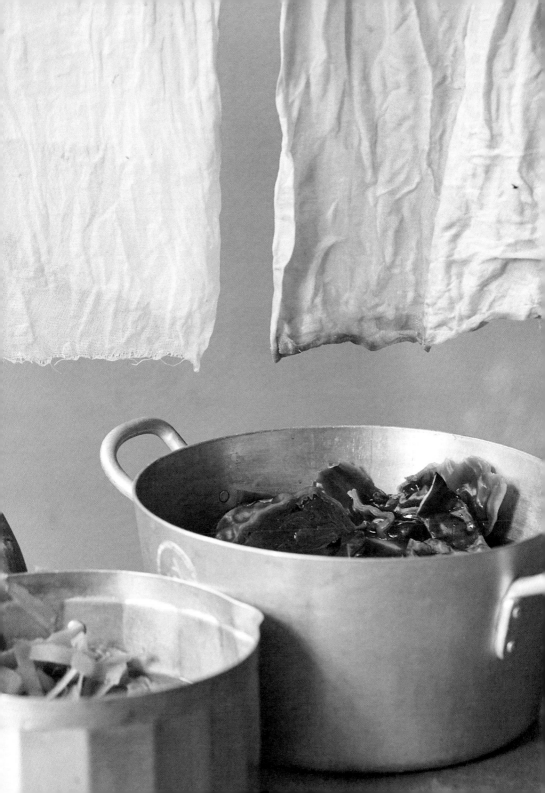

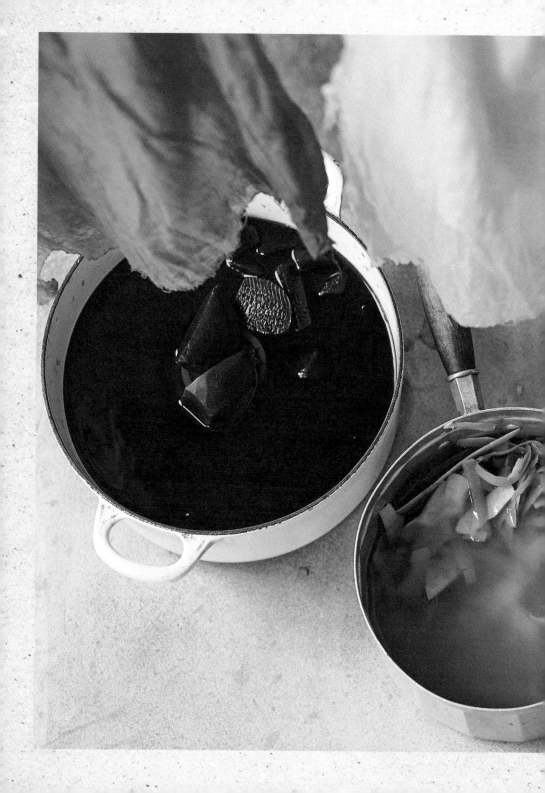

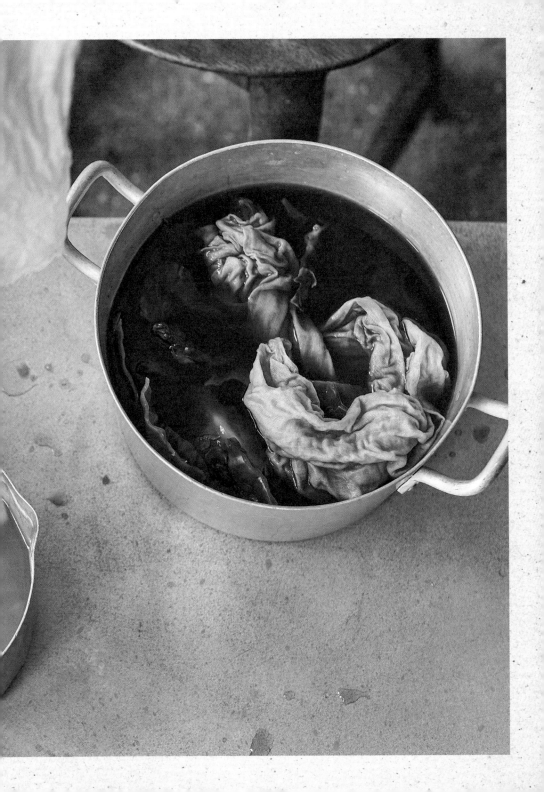

LEMON-PEEL
TOILET DROPS

**MAKES APPROX. 80 ML
(3 FL OZ)**

INGREDIENTS:

1 tablespoon bicarbonate of soda
  (baking soda)
4 tablespoons white wine vinegar
2 tablespoons vodka
15 drops of Lemon Peel Oil *(see
  page 134)*

YOU WILL NEED:

spray bottle or a bottle with
  a pipette

TIP:

*Always label your homemade
products clearly and keep them
out of reach of children and pets.*

I've been in more than my fair share of embarrassing situations in my life, across all possible categories. It's for this reason that I try to make my home a place where guests have everything they might need to avoid unfortunate situations! A small bottle of toilet drops in the bathroom is a perfect example. Using a few drops in the toilet bowl before doing what you need to do helps to neutralise odours. Here, we make a lemon peel oil to create the toilet drops.

01 To start, make your own homemade lemon peel oil by following the instructions on page 134.

02 In a mixing bowl, combine the bicarbonate of soda, vinegar and vodka. The mixture will fizz a bit. Stir gently until it's well combined and the fizzing subsides.

03 Add your lemon peel oil and stir thoroughly to ensure the oil is evenly distributed. Carefully transfer the mixture into either a spray bottle or a bottle with a pipette.

04 These drops will keep for 6 months but are their most effective within the first 3.

05 Shake well before each use. To use, add about 5 drops to the toilet bowl after flushing.

THE WHY:

• This lemon oil not only has a pleasant fragrance, but also has natural deodorising properties.

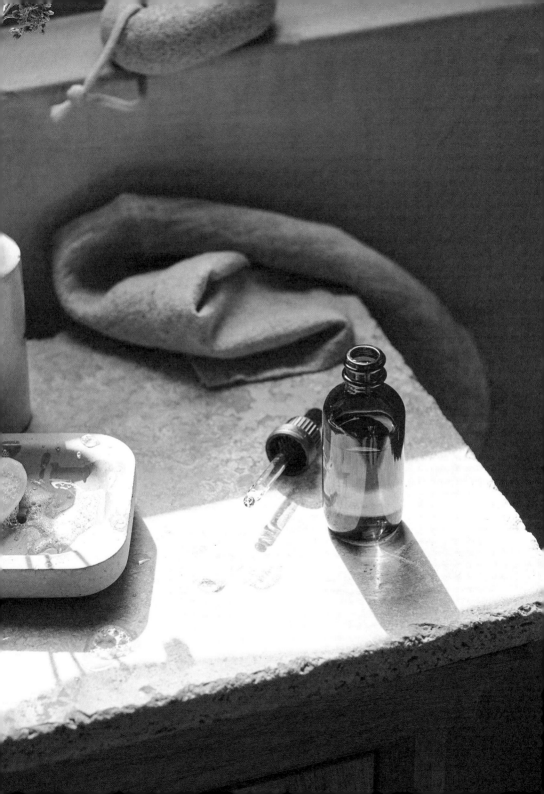

APPLE CORE HAND SANITISER

MAKES APPROX. 75 ML (3 FL OZ)

INGREDIENTS:

5–6 apple cores *(if you're the only apple-eater in your household, you can freeze them as you go until you've got enough, then just thaw on the day you plan to make the sanitiser)*

4 tablespoons high-proof vodka or isopropyl alcohol *(at least 70 per cent alcohol content)*

1 tablespoon aloe vera gel *(see page 139 for how to extract aloe gel from a leaf)*

5–6 drops of tea tree essential oil

YOU WILL NEED:

glass jar or bottle with a secure lid
fine-mesh strainer
small bowl
small glass bottle with a pump

The skin around my eyes and on my hands is prone to eczema, and my hands have never got on well with the average hand sanitiser you might find on the market. I'm not an everyday hand-sanitiser-type, but at a music festival or when I'm doing a lot of public transport travelling, I'll be sure to take a bottle of this.

01 First, remove any seeds or stems from your apple cores. Chop the cores into smaller pieces or give them a very quick whizz in a blender.

02 Place the chopped apple cores in a clean glass jar or bottle and cover them with the vodka or isopropyl alcohol. Make sure the alcohol completely covers the apple core pieces. Seal the jar or bottle tightly with a lid.

03 Allow the apple core pieces to steep in the alcohol for at least 24 hours. During this time, the alcohol will extract the antimicrobial compounds from the apple cores.

04 When you're ready, strain the liquid through a fine-mesh strainer into a clean bowl. Squeeze the apple cores to extract as much liquid as possible. Compost the leftover cores.

05 Add the aloe vera gel and tea tree oil to the mixture in the bowl and stir well. Transfer into a reusable glass bottle with a pump.

06 To use, apply a small amount of the apple core hand sanitiser to your hands and rub them together until dry.

THE WHY:

- Apples contain natural antimicrobial compounds, such as malic acid, which can help reduce the number of germs on your hands. The apple cores' natural sugars and water content help to hydrate and moisturise the skin, preventing the dryness that often occurs with commercial hand sanitisers. The aloe vera will add extra moisture, while the tea tree oil has additional antibacterial properties and gives a pleasant scent.

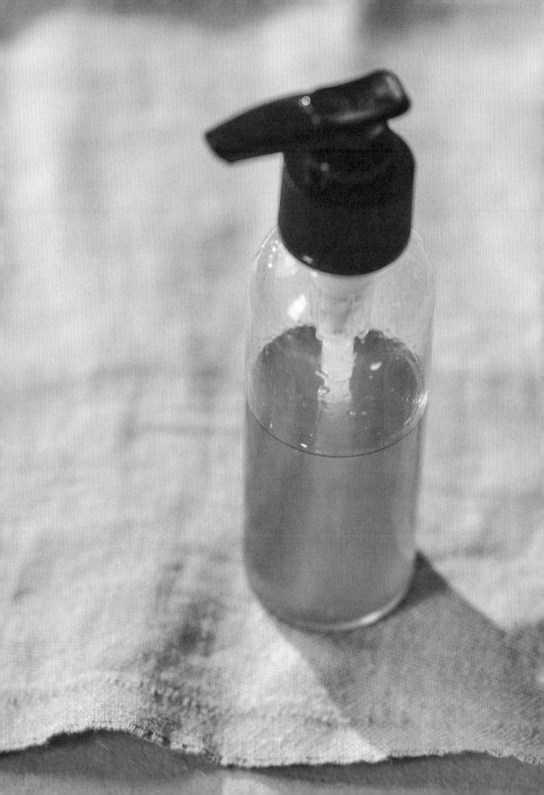

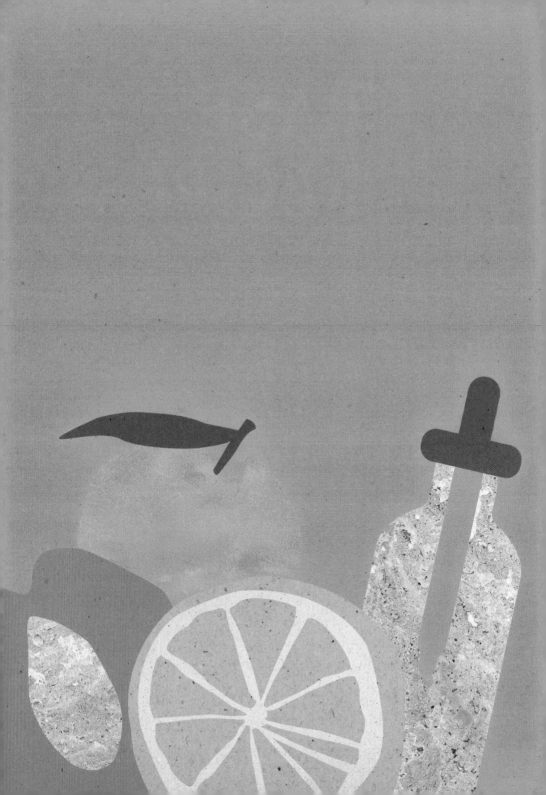

BASE RECIPES

Each oil that I explain how to create in this book is an infusion as opposed to an essential oil. But what's the difference? The two approaches, while rooted in harnessing the benefits of plants, differ significantly in their preparation, potency, and application. Essential oils are extracted through distillation. They're more concentrated and potent than infusions and thus a lot more of the plant is needed to make an essential oil. Their potency requires cautious handling, and whilst a few essential oils can be applied directly to the skin, most require dilution in a carrier oil to ensure safe usage.

On the other hand, infusions offer a gentler, more accessible route to harnessing the benefits of plants. They're a much more realistic and practical option for creating at home, they can be crafted simply by filling a jar with fresh or dried herbs, then covering them with a carrier oil, like olive or almond oil. Over the course of around a month, these oils meld with the plant material, gradually extracting oil-soluble constituents, including traces of essential oils. Infusions, often used as stand-alone treatments or as foundations for skincare products, penetrate the skin naturally, carrying the plant's essence deeper into the body.

MINT-INFUSED OIL

INGREDIENTS:

wilted mint leaves *(as many as you have)*
almond oil, olive oil or other carrier oil of your choice

YOU WILL NEED:

pestle and mortar *(if you don't have these, a spoon will do)*
airtight container with a lid *(like a Kilner jar)*
fine-mesh strainer or muslin *(cheesecloth)*
small bottle

TIP:

If you'd like to increase the potency next time you make this, simply repeat the above steps using the same quantity of oil but more leaves.

We haven't given precise measurements here, as it depends on how many mint leaves you have to use up, so you can make as much or as little as you wish.

01 Make sure your mint leaves are dry. Use a pestle and mortar (or the back of a spoon against a hard, solid surface) to crush the leaves. The idea is to mash but not mangle them; you're aiming to unlock their aromatic essence, but not turn them to paste!

02 Transfer the crushed mint into the jar, then pour over enough carrier oil to cover them. The amount of carrier oil you use to steep your leaves will determine how much infused oil you ultimately end up with. Shake the jar a little to make sure all the leaves are submerged.

03 Seal the lid and leave the jar to sit in a warm, dark place for 24–48 hours.

04 After this, strain the leaves from the liquid using a fine-mesh strainer or a piece of muslin (cheesecloth). If there are any leaf remnants in the oil, try to remove them by hand, or strain again. Your oil will last longer with as few bits as possible left in it. Transfer the strained oil to a bottle.

05 The oil is now ready to be used in the Wilted Mint Lip Balm on page 30. This oil will keep for 3–6 months in a cool, dry place.

GINGER OIL

MAKES APPROX. 30ML OF OIL

INGREDIENTS:

7 tablespoons coconut oil
2–3 pieces of fresh root ginger
(approx. 100 g (3½ oz)), chopped

YOU WILL NEED:

saucepan
fine-mesh strainer
small bottle or jar

In this book we'll use this infusion in a shampoo bar (see page 40), but there are other ways you can incorporate this into your own creations. It can be applied as a spot treatment, you can use a few drops in a facial toner or mix some into a face mask! Its top benefit is increasing the radiance of the skin. It does this by boosting circulation, boosting collagen production and working to even out skin tone.

01 Melt the coconut oil in a small saucepan over a very low heat. Once melted, it should be enough to cover the base.

02 Add the chopped ginger and stir to ensure it's coated in the oil, then leave for 40 minutes to infuse, still over the very low heat. You're aiming to warm it, but not cook it. Stir occasionally.

03 Remove from the heat and allow to cool before straining, then decant into a bottle or jar. Your oil is now ready to use in our Ginger Shampoo Bar (see page 40).

LEMON PEEL OIL

MAKES 75 ML (3 FL OZ) OIL

INGREDIENTS:

peel of 4–6 lemons, finely grated
75–100 ml (2½–3½ fl oz) olive oil

YOU WILL NEED:

heatproof bowl and saucepan
  to create a bain-marie/
  double-boiler
fine-mesh strainer
tinted glass bottle

For me, the biggest appeal of lemon oil is its fresh scent. You'll find lemon in so many home cleaning, laundry and deodorising products for this reason, but it's not this oil's only plus point. Lemon can help remove limescale, it's naturally antibacterial and antiseptic, it helps to break down grease and can also reduce or remove stains. It's a safe bet to include lemon oil in pretty much any cleaning, fabric or homecare formula!

01 Fill the saucepan with about 5 cm (2 in) water and bring to a simmer over medium heat. Place the heatproof bowl on top of the saucepan, ensuring it fits securely without touching the water.

02 Add the lemon peel and oil to the bowl and stir to combine. Leave to infuse over the heat for 30 minutes– 1 hour, stirring occasionally, until the smell of lemons completely replaces the smell of olive oil. You may need to top up the water in the pan now and then.

03 When your lemon peel oil is ready, remove from the heat and allow to cool, before straining the oil to remove the peel. Decant the infused oil into a bottle. It is now ready to be used in the Lemon Peel Toilet Drops (page 126) recipe. The oil will last for 6 months if stored appropriately in a cool place, out of direct sunlight.

ORANGE PEEL OIL

**MAKES 75–100 ML
(3–3½ FL OZ)**

INGREDIENTS:

finely grated peel of 4–6 oranges
75–100 ml *(2½–3½ fl oz)* olive oil

YOU WILL NEED:

heatproof bowl and saucepan to
   create a bain-marie/double-boiler
fine-mesh strainer
tinted glass bottle with 100 ml
   (3½ fl oz) capacity

Following the same logic as I've just mentioned for lemon peel oil, I've matched orange oil with a deodorant recipe in this book. It's great at odour neutralising! It boasts similar benefits to lemon, but is less potent and therefore less likely to irritate your skin. Hence, lemon has been prioritised for home recipes and orange can work wonders in skin products when properly diluted.

01 Fill the saucepan with about 5 cm (2 in) water and bring to a simmer over medium heat. Place the heatproof bowl on top of the saucepan, ensuring it fits securely without touching the water.

02 Add the orange peel and oil to the bowl and stir to combine. Leave to infuse over the heat for 30 minutes–1 hour, stirring occasionally, until the smell of oranges completely replaces the smell of olive oil. You may need to top up the water in the pan now and then.

03 When your orange peel oil is ready, remove from the heat and allow to cool, before straining the oil to remove the peel. Decant the infused oil into a bottle. It is now ready to be used in the body oil on page 60. This infusion will keep for 6 months if stored appropriately, away from heat and direct sunlight.

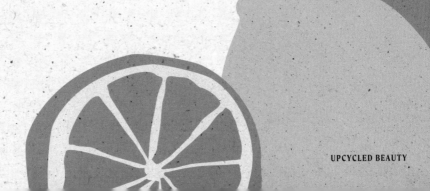

APRICOT KERNEL OIL

**MAKES APPROX. 10ML
(¹/₃ FL OZ) OF OIL**

INGREDIENTS:

apricot kernels from 1 punnet of
fruit (approx. 8)

YOU WILL NEED:

jar with a lid or small amber or
blue glass bottle

If you've been enjoying a punnet of apricots, keep the stones!
Encased within them is the seed, more commonly known as the
kernel, and this is what we'll make our oil from.

01 Pop all the kernels into a food processor and blend until
you have a fine powder. Tip the powder into a large
mixing bowl and add 2 tablespoons of warm water.

02 Begin to knead. Continue kneading, adding another
tablespoon of warm water about every minute over the
course of 5 minutes. The dough should change in nature
to feel sticky and oily. Resist the urge to add too much
water – the dough should never feel wet.

03 After several minutes of kneading, you'll notice the
dough will start to feel oily. Do not add any more water
at this point, just begin squeezing the dough, and oil
should come from it. You can squeeze directly from the
dough into your chosen oil container (we recommend
an amber or blue glass bottle), or you can strain it first,
if needed.

04 The oil should keep for up to 6 months if stored in a
cool, dry place. It's ready to be used in our Apricot
Hand Cream (see page 32).

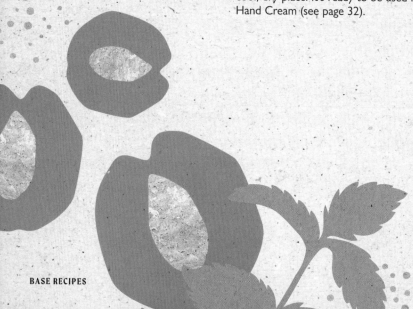

CINNAMON OIL

MAKES APPROX. 50 ML

INGREDIENTS:

10 clean, dry cinnamon sticks
avocado oil (about 50 ml (2 fl oz)

YOU WILL NEED:

jar with a lid or small tinted bottle

At UpCircle we use upcycled cinnamon bark in our perfume.
The oil created from it is spicy and peppery with a blush of vanilla
and we source it from Sri Lanka. The sun-warmed cinnamon bark
curls into quills on drying, but less uniform rolls are left behind.
The spice market's loss is our gain as these imperfect quills are
distilled into a sweet, woody oil that has a sophisticated and
elegant scent.

01 Pop the cinnamon sticks into your jar and fill the jar
with enough avocado oil to cover the sticks. Leave in a
sunny spot for 3–5 weeks. Shake the jar a little daily.

02 When it's ready, strain the oil, discard the cinnamon
sticks and pour the oil into a clean bottle. It is now
ready to use in the Plumping Cinnamon Lip Oil (see
page 58).

03 It will keep for 6 months if stored appropriately,
away from heat and direct sunlight.

BEETROOT POWDER

MAKES ABOUT 100 G (3½ OZ) OF POWDER

INGREDIENTS:

2–3 beetroots

Beetroot is my mum's favourite vegetable and she grows it at home. Unfortunately, I'd be lying if I said it was in my top 15 vegetables, so when she brings me a load over, it's usually turned into powder to avoid it being wasted! Sorry, Mum.

01 Wash your beetroots thoroughly, then grate them or use a food processor to finely dice them.

02 Spread them out on a baking tray lined with baking paper (parchment paper) and leave on a sunny windowsill for at least 48 hours. Alternatively, place in the oven set to a very low heat (about 100°C/210°F/ gas ¼) and leave to dehydrate for about 20 minutes. Toss the contents of the tray, then return to the oven for an additional 20 minutes. You'll know they're ready when they are crispy. The aim is to remove all the moisture.

03 Once ready, transfer the dried-out beetroot to a coffee grinder or blender and grind until you have a fine powder with a beautiful pink hue. If stored appropriately in an air-tight container in a cool dry place, your powder should last a year.

04 Use in our Beetroot Cheek Tint (see page 88).

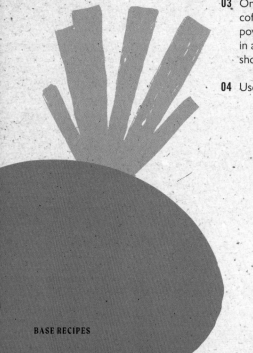

HOW TO EXTRACT ALOE VERA GEL FROM THE LEAF

While you can purchase aloe vera gel pretty easily, extracting it from a leaf is a straightforward process. Here's a step-by-step guide on how to do this yourself.

01 Select a mature and healthy leaf from the outermost part of the aloe vera plant. The outer leaves are usually larger and more robust, making them better for harvesting.

02 Rinse the aloe vera leaf thoroughly under running water to remove any dirt, debris or potential pesticides or chemicals.

03 Using a sharp knife or scissors, cut the leaf close to the base of the plant. Aim for a clean cut, as jagged edges can make it more challenging to extract the gel later on.

04 Once you've cut the leaf, you may notice a yellowish substance oozing out. This is the latex, which can have a bitter taste and may cause skin irritation in some people. To remove the latex, place the cut leaf upright in a container or on an incline with the cut side down. Allow it to drain for 10–15 minutes.

05 After draining the latex, place the leaf flat on a chopping board. Using a knife, carefully cut off the serrated edges and slice off the top layer of the leaf's skin (the green outer layer) on both sides. Be gentle and cautious, taking care not to cut too deep, as you want to preserve the gel beneath the skin.

06 Once you've removed the skin, you'll see the clear gel underneath. Using a spoon or a butter knife, carefully scoop out the gel from the leaf. Be gentle to avoid damaging the gel or incorporating any bits of the leaf's skin.

07 Collect the extracted gel in a clean bowl or container. You can use it immediately or store it in an airtight container in the refrigerator for future use. It will keep for 2–3 weeks.

INDEX

ABOUT ANNA

Anna was only 22 years old when she launched UpCircle, the brand that's now the UK's #1 upcycled beauty brand. Stocked in over 50 countries, UpCircle's vast and rapidly growing product range spans an impressive 50+ upcycled ingredients.

Founders tend to wear a lot of hats, but Anna loosely describes her role within the brand as 'The Story-Teller'. She heads up the marketing and warehouse teams for UpCircle and is the brand's voice whenever it requires one. Pitches, panels, podcasts, press interviews, awards, radio, TV appearances – all Anna. Aside from the themes of beauty and the circular economy, Anna keeps a personal target to speak on the subject of women in business once a week.

By age 27, Anna was named as one of Forbes 30 Under 30 honourees. She credits her success to a willingness to roll up her sleeves and get involved in any task that requires it, and her ability to find humour to any situation, no matter how calamitous it may seem! Anna's work at the intersection of beauty, entrepreneurship, circular innovation and climate change demonstrates that she is a key leader in the sustainability space.

ACKNOWLEDGMENTS

First and foremost, I'd like to thank William. We're siblings by chance but business partners by choice and there's no way any of this would have happened without his brain or his unwavering dedication to UpCircle's success. I've always known that he's the smartest person I know, but his irritatingly good instincts in the world of skincare and beauty have certainly been a surprise! I'm so proud of us as a duo and what we've created, so thanks for halving the stress of it all with me.

Second, I'd like to acknowledge the rest of the Brightmans. Whether it's collecting coffee during the festive season, labelling up unexpected huge wholesale orders, driving us to trade shows and helping us sell over countless weekends, or modelling for us – my sisters and parents are the best support system William and I could possibly ask for!

Next Marcus and Maya, my family. Marcus you are the love of my life. You're my motivation and my motivator and I'm so glad I have you.

I'd also like to thank the book team for guiding me through this process and for bringing my ideas to life visually. Issy, Nikki, Lizzie and Libby you're all so incredibly talented and I couldn't have asked for a better team to highlight the beauty of upcycling.

Finally, to the UpCircle team. You guys are UpCircle. Thank you all for your passion, your wit, your grit, your willingness to get stuck in (like being the models in this book) and for everything you do to make this brand of ours what it is.

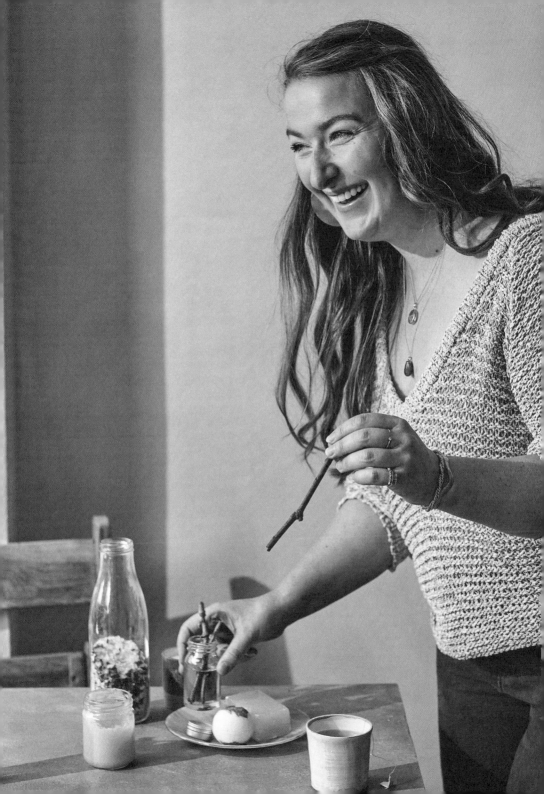

Published in 2024 by Hardie Grant Books,
an imprint of Hardie Grant Publishing

Hardie Grant Books (London)
5th & 6th Floors
52–54 Southwark Street
London SE1 1UN

Hardie Grant Books (Melbourne)
Building 1, 658 Church Street
Richmond, Victoria 3121

hardiegrantbooks.com

All rights reserved. No part of this publication may be reproduced, stored in a retrieval system
or transmitted in any form by any means, electronic, mechanical, photocopying, recording or
otherwise, without the prior written permission of the publishers and copyright holders.

The moral rights of the author have been asserted.

Copyright text © Anna Brightman
Copyright photography © Lizzie Mayson

British Library Cataloguing-in-Publication Data. A catalogue record
for this book is available from the British Library.

UpCycled Beauty
978-178488-733-9

10 9 8 7 6 5 4 3 2 1

Publishing Director: Kajal Mistry
Commissioning Editor: Isabel Gonzalez-Prendergast
Copyeditor: Tara O'Sullivan
Food & Prop Stylist: Libby Silbermann
Photographer: Lizzie Mayson
Design & Illustration: Studio Nic & Lou
Production Controller: Martina Georgieva

Colour reproduction by p2d
Printed and bound in China by Leo Paper Products Ltd.

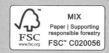